Jill Florence Lackey, PhD

Accountability in Social Services
The Culture of the Paper Program

Pre-publication
REVIEWS,
COMMENTARIES,
EVALUATIONS . . .

"Through the use of case examples, Dr. Lackey describes how social service programs can exist on paper only; that is, through formal reports documenting that they are providing what they ought, while in reality supplying none or almost none of the services they were funded to provide. She skillfully uses theory to explain how the lack of accountability at many levels—potential consumers, funding sources, program evaluators, and the sponsoring organization—often leads to 'paper programs.' She goes further to describe how individuals and organizations manage to avoid becoming paper programs, by strengthening accountability and developing an ethical, consumer-focused culture.

This book is particularly helpful for graduate students in the social sciences and in human services management. Dr. Lackey is courageously honest in sharing her own co-optation experiences as an evaluator of paper programs. Although her experiences will sound painfully familiar to many seasoned evaluators, they provide important warnings for students and newly minted administrators and evaluation staff. Her willingness to step back and review her many years of evaluation experience in a theoretical context is both fresh and useful.

In particular, I appreciate her review of the accountability problems associated with community coalitions. Although coalitions have become an intensely popular strategy for addressing entrenched social maladies, they are uniquely burdened by planning and decision-making problems. This book addresses the concept of 'culture conflicts' when bringing disparate groups to the coalition table, and the need for considerable care and feeding of the coalition, to the detriment of any actual service delivery. It also provides useful insights into the role of the media, and why it does not play more of a watchdog role in public programs."

Denise Dion Hallfors, PhD
Senior Research Scientist,
Pacific Institute for Research
and Evaluation (PIRE)

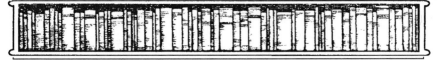

More pre-publication
REVIEWS, COMMENTARIES, EVALUATIONS . . .

"**D**r. Lackey's book *Accountability in Social Services* provides an insightful and engaging series of case studies of local social service programs from the perspective of a practicing "ground-level" program evaluator.

The existence of paper programs is placed in the theoretical context of Bourdieu's theory of practice and habitus, as well as Gramsci's theory of hegemony. The postmodernist critique that the real is increasingly replaced by a 'representation of the real,' a virtual reality, is also incorporated in the analysis. Thus the analysis is placed in a larger theoretical context, which will be of interest to academically inclined audiences. However, this book is written in an engaging, concise, and accessible style that will make it of interest and value to a very broad audience.

While the emphasis is on the paper program and the related issues of structural lack of real accountability, the paper programs are compared to the (more prevalent) set of well-implemented and effective programs which the author has also evaluated. Using this comparative case study approach, Dr. Lackey concludes that the primary factors that can reduce the number of paper programs are ethical leadership and staff, increased consumerism, and better structural and financial separation of evaluation from dependence on the program being evaluated.

This book will be of interest to a broad range of academic and applied audiences. The chapter on coalitions—which may become ends in themselves—is particularly interesting, given the current emphasis in health and human services on partnerships and coalitions. In particular, applied audiences in eval-uation, social services, social work, and policy analysis will find this book relevant. Academics who study the sociology of organizations, administrative science, social welfare policy, and political science will also find this an intriguing source of grounded data and analysis."

D. Paul Moberg, PhD
Deputy Director and Senior Scientist,
University of Wisconsin
Population Health Institute

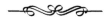

"**D**r. Lackey, an evaluator of social programs, finds that many of the programs she is called upon to study do not exist, not in terms of real service to real people. The programs are paper illusions—brochures, applications, and reports. Yet they keep getting funded. She attributes the victory of 'paper' over reality to the lack of influence exerted by the programs' putative monitors: clients, national organizations, funders, and evaluators, each of which is hobbled by characteristics of the system. The author's purpose here is to alert all actors in the social service world to the dysfunctions that afflict the system and to spur greater accountability. A book well worth reading and taking seriously."

Carol H. Weiss, PhD
Beatrice B. Whiting Research Professor
of Education,
Harvard Graduate School of Education

More pre-publication
REVIEWS, COMMENTARIES, EVALUATIONS . . .

"*Accountability in Social Services* is highly recommended reading for anyone associated with funding social programs, including legislators, government officials, foundation members, and businesses. It also provides valuable information for persons who are developing and implementing social programs or those who are charged with evaluating these programs. Members of the media may also discover their responsibility to the general public to reveal the real story behind social programs in their communities.

Dr. Lackey skillfully makes a case for the importance of accountability at all levels of social programming from the customers it is designed to assist, through the funding source and program evaluators to the program's sponsoring organization. She uses case studies of actual programs to demonstrate the importance of accountability from the development of the program through implementation to evaluation. It is Dr. Lackey's contention that a lack of accountability has led to the development of 'paper programs'—programs that look good on paper but that do not deliver what they promise. Paper programs may receive millions of dollars in funding without providing a fraction of the services promised because accountability systems often are inadequate, underfunded, or ignored in the process of development and implementation. Dr. Lackey identifies glaring gaps in the evaluation process that can allow paper programs to exist. On the other hand, accountability systems can help to draw attention to successful programs and help to keep them funded. I recommend this book for anyone involved in social services programs."

Denise J. Brandon, PhD
Associate Professor,
University of Tennessee Extension

The Haworth Press
New York • London • Oxford

Accountability in Social Services
The Culture of the Paper Program

HAWORTH Health and Social Policy
Marvin D. Feit, PhD

Accountability in Social Services
The Culture of the Paper Program

Jill Florence Lackey, PhD

The Haworth Press
New York • London • Oxford

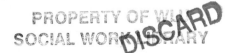

For more information on this book or to order, visit
http://www.haworthpress.com/store/product.asp?sku=5556

or call 1-800-HAWORTH (800-429-6784) in the United States and Canada
or (607) 722-5857 outside the United States and Canada

or contact orders@HaworthPress.com

The Haworth Press, Inc., 10 Alice Street, Binghamton, NY 13904-1580.

PUBLISHER'S NOTES
The development, preparation, and publication of this work has been undertaken with great care. However, the Publisher, employees, editors, and agents of The Haworth Press are not responsible for any errors contained herein or for consequences that may ensue from use of materials or information contained in this work. The Haworth Press is committed to the dissemination of ideas and information according to the highest standards of intellectual freedom and the free exchange of ideas. Statements made and opinions expressed in this publication do not necessarily reflect the views of the Publisher, Directors, management, or staff of The Haworth Press, Inc., or an endorsement by them.

Identities and circumstances of individuals and organizations discussed in this book have been changed to protect anonymity and confidentiality.

Cover design by Laurie J. Steelman.

Library of Congress Cataloging-in-Publication Data

Lackey, Jill Florence.
    Accountability in social services : the culture of the paper program / Jill Florence Lackey.
        p. cm.
    Includes bibliographical references and index.
    ISBN-13: 978-0-7890-2374-2 (hard : alk. paper)
    ISBN-10: 0-7890-2374-1 (hard : alk. paper)
    ISBN-13: 978-0-7890-2375-9 (soft : alk. paper)
    ISBN-10: 0-7890-2375-X (soft : alk. paper)
    1. Social service—United States—Evaluation.
[DNLM: 1. Social Work. 2. Program Evaluation.] I. Title.

HV91.L14 2006
361.3068'4—dc22

        2005024405

Dedicated to my late mother, Joy Lackey,
who convinced me I had the courage to write this book

ABOUT THE AUTHOR

Jill Florence Lackey, PhD, a cultural anthropologist, is founder and director of Jill Florence Lackey & Associates and of Urban Anthropology Inc. (UrbAn), the only nonprofit organization in the United States engaged exclusively in the practice of urban anthropology. She teaches anthropology and evaluation research at Marquette University's College of Professional Studies in Milwaukee, Wisconsin. Dr. Lackey's work has appeared in a variety of publications, including *Evaluation Practice, Human Organization, Practicing Anthropology, Evaluation and Program Planning,* and *Anthropology News.*

CONTENTS

Preface

My goal in writing this book was clearly not the denigration of social services. Social services are absolutely needed in our society—particularly by the most vulnerable members of the population. My ultimate goal was to present information that might result in more funded services actually reaching their targets. This work assesses problems in accountability mechanisms at most levels of the social service delivery system and demonstrates ways that lack of accountability sometimes results in services not reaching their targets. I am quite aware that systems other than social services can and do lack these accountability mechanisms. Enron is one case in point. However, the social service delivery system is a topic I happen to know a great deal about, being an evaluator specializing in it.

It took me years to decide to write this book. I would not describe myself as a risk taker or as someone who invites controversy. In fact, I would describe myself as a relative coward. Curiously, it was my now-departed mother who actually told me I had to write this book—and we do tend to obey our mothers, even in middle age. I had deep concerns that the work would be misrepresented or used as a way to deny funding for social services. I worried that some might interpret the book as creating concerns over the existence of social services rather than creating concerns about these services reaching the consumers and communities they are supposed to help. I also wondered if anyone would ever engage my firm in evaluation again, for fear that their pet project might make it into another volume as an example of a "paper program"—no matter how well disguised the program might be in the narrative.

This work is based on case studies of over fifty program evaluations that my research firm has conducted. The book is designed to present information not on actual outcomes from these evaluations, but rather on the implementation process these programs used or failed to use and how these processes reflect and feed back into larger structures within the society. The book shows how the growing cultural

doi:10.1300/5556_a

trend of accepting representation of a reality as the reality itself plays into lack of accountability—hence the subtitle, *The Culture of the Paper Program.*

This work also highlights some of the nearly heroic efforts of staff within social service programs and how these staff set precedents for solid program delivery within their organizations. The efforts of these workers unfolded despite having almost no accountability mechanisms in place, and some of these efforts continued for decades. However, I was very saddened to learn that a number of the staff highlighted in this book have left their programs in the year between submitting this manuscript and publication. At this time, I do not know the reasons why they left their positions, but it is a topic I intend to investigate in future research.

Acknowledgments

I would like to extend special thanks to those researchers who read this manuscript and provided feedback, including Alice Kehoe and Mary Roffers.

I would also like to thank the scores of people in my personal network of friends and extended family that heard of my intention to write this book and gave me many accounts of their own experiences with the social service delivery system—both best practices and sometimes the opposite. In many cases, these accounts convinced me of the need for this book and strengthened my drive to write it. Among these scores of people I include Judy Conti, Mary Harris, Ralph Dietrich, Jacqueline Ward, Latrelle Davis, Susan Andrews, David Florence, and above all my always principled mother, Joy Lackey.

doi:10.1300/5556_b

Chapter 1

Introducing the Paper Program

What are "paper programs," and how do they emerge in the social service delivery system? As the name implies, paper programs are those that exist, for the most part, on paper only. They are programs whose formal documents (e.g., grant proposals, public relations material, reports to funding agencies) specify the services or other resources they are supposed to provide, and their routine documentation suggests they are providing what they claim, but in reality the programs are providing none or a mere fraction of these services. The argument that this book consistently makes is that paper programs can exist because of the lack of accountability mechanisms among groups and cultural institutions with stakes in the social service delivery system—from the consumers of services, to funding agencies, to the taxpayers, to sponsoring organizations, to program evaluators, to the media. The book argues that although demands for accountability have actually increased over the past decades through government and private mandates (Martin & Kettner, 1997), nearly all monitoring in this system is done through written communication. Only rarely does face-to-face interaction occur. For purposes of accountability, paper reports in essence become the program.

To some, the concept of a paper program may seem incredible. Social services are organized responses to difficult, usually enduring, social problems that are most often experienced by vulnerable individuals—individuals who become the consumers or clients of the programs. Studies on excellence in social service organizations reveal that one of the dimensions of excellence reported most often by organizational leaders is orientation to serving client needs (Harvey, 1998; Rapp & Poertner, 1992). According to Manning (2003), social or human service organizations have unique callings: "First, people are the raw material of the organization. Second, human service

doi:10.1300/5556_01

organizations are mandated to promote and protect the welfare of the people they serve" (p. 22). Through a series of case studies, I argue that this orientation toward clients does occur frequently—especially where ethics-based staff have strong voices in program operations—but in daily practice, complex processes throughout the system tend to divert attention from the stated ideal, and almost nothing exists in the system to refocus the effort. The argument that the ideal does exist should be what surprises the reader in the upcoming chapters rather than the uncovering of paper programs, because the cultural milieu in which most social programs operate does so little to encourage an orientation toward the usually vulnerable consumers of service.

This book describes processes that occur at the program level, the level of the social service delivery system, and beyond. At the program level, most staff profess the ideal of commitment to clients, but the actual required work and the accountability obligations tend to center on printed products rather than client-staff relations. This mismatch between expressed ideals and routine practices is a centerpiece of Bourdieu's (1977) theory of practice. Bourdieu argued that embedded practices and dispositions, rather than stated ideals, tend to guide human behavior. These dispositions and patterns of practice emerge through historical and adaptive processes, but over time the factors that led to these practices may be forgotten and the practices continue with minimal human reflection—a phenomenon Bourdieu termed *habitus*. Individuals find themselves submerged in habitual and officially approved practices, and while some may not always follow the patterns, they nevertheless appear natural over time.

One routine activity that has increased in postmodern times is the practice of replacing the real with a representation of the real (Baudrillard, 1994). In many cases, paper reports as opposed to actual transactions are used to "prove" that something exists, which occurs often with social programs. Funding sources for programs usually require written reports of program operations and expenditures, but funding personnel seldom conduct site visits to determine whether these services are actually provided. This has become a virtual reality of accountability mechanisms. On their end, program personnel invest a great deal of time and energy in the creation of these paper products, diverting energy from the actual objectives of the program. The documentation is often necessary for communicating with other staff, maintaining a history of what services or resources have been provided (sometimes just to jog the memory), and obviously because no one can be present to monitor every transaction—the documentation is the next best thing. The problems begin to arise when the representation of the transaction becomes the proof of the transaction, and ultimately when it replaces the transaction itself. The history is written and the created image is treated like the final reified commodity (Jameson, 1984).

Local practices do not emerge in a vacuum. Social programs are embedded in systems that include groups ranging from the least powerful consumers of services to very powerful government and capitalist interests. Social services may not be a high priority for the more powerful interests, and the process of merely securing financial backing for the programs involves hegemonic relationships. The theory of hegemony derives from the recognition that government and other dominant interests cannot enforce control over any subordinate groups without these groups yielding a limited consent (Gramsci, 1971). Gramsci, like the Marxists, focused on class relations, while rejecting the determinism and economism of the Marxists. He added a psychocultural dimension where human agency and subordinate formations play roles in the development of policies and ideologies. According to this approach, dominant groups in capitalist societies rule through power blocs, or special-purpose alliances. The alliances may include groups that negotiate their limited consent in return for getting some of their interests represented in the power bloc—a process called *co-optation*. These blocs are historical and as such, are fluid coalitions of interests that share political solidarity at some shifting point in time. They often represent groups from several classes.

Social service organizations and advocacy groups find their way into these alliances. For example, social service agencies may receive funding to treat individuals for what are really complex, difficult, and enduring social problems. The problems may include poverty, crime, child abuse, homelessness, hunger, alcohol, and illegal drugs—problems more often faced by those in the lower socioeconomic strata than by those in the upper. Although these problems can easily be ignored by the more powerful members of the blocs, they need some form of limited consent from subordinate groups to rule. Hence, through processes of interpenetration and mixing, subordinate groups with some interests at odds with those of dominant groups may actually invade hegemony (Canclini, 1995). As conceptualized, hegemony is a seat of struggle and also a venue for change.

Through the case studies in the upcoming chapters, my hope is that the reader will be able to follow the ways that hegemonic relationships can result in the basic existence of social programs, the creation of ideologies about social programs through sources such as the mass media, and also the weak incentives for holding social programs accountable. However, this venue for change argued by some of the less deterministic hegemony theorists is one of the major points of optimism in this book as well, and is addressed in the concluding chapter.

This book is based on my own evaluation and research consultant work with over fifty social programs and experience in directing two nonprofit organizations. Many of these social programs are highlighted in the upcoming chapters, although specific names and other identifiers have been altered. The work focuses on case studies of programs, their implementation, and the monitoring mechanisms that were and were not in place during program operations. Again, it is my hope that the reader experiences surprise at the information provided—not because of the information on paper programs, but because of the information on extraordinary social service efforts (and their staff) that continue on and on with so little out there to ensure their performance and, for that matter, their survival.

Chapter 2

Varieties of Paper Programs

There are, of course, varying degrees of paper programs. These range from out-and-out fraud to programs that are locked into paper processes. The following example of the "program in a box" represents the more extreme end of the continuum. I will later discuss the more common variety.

PAY: THE PROGRAM IN A BOX

I was exposed to the "PAY" program years before I became its evaluator (PAY is an acronym for Positive Alternatives for Youth). I attended an adolescent programming conference in the early 1990s, and during a workshop a well-prepared team of two men and two women were discussing what appeared to be an innovative demonstration project. The team (which I learned later was the program staff) explained that PAY had been planned as an alternative aftercare program for 120 youths who had spent over six months in residential treatment centers for law offenses, substance abuse, or other problem behaviors.

The team claimed that conventional aftercare programming in the area usually only included counseling, while their project offered positive alternatives to the delinquent lifestyle, either through direct services or through monitored referrals. These alternatives could include recreational programs, volunteer opportunities with stipends, job training and placement, special interest clubs, client support groups, and family social activities, as well as the more conventional case management and counseling services.

To illustrate their innovations, the team presented a video of the PAY Opportunities Fair they held early in the program's first year.

doi:10.1300/5556_02

5

The video showed hundreds of youths listening to presentations on program options and being interviewed by allied organizational representatives who offered them opportunities to participate in sports leagues, job training programs, and summer camps. After the video, the team said that PAY was in its last year of a three-year grant and was well on its way to becoming a model for opportunity-based programming.

One year later, I received a telephone call from a high-level administrator of PAY's parent organization, the "City Life Institute." The administrator told me that PAY was now out of operation because the three-year demonstration grant had ended, but they needed an evaluation. Unfortunately, the program's first evaluator had failed to produce a report and the federal funding agency was demanding one. Could I come in and evaluate this effort retrospectively?

We met. During our discussion, the administrator explained that he knew less than he should about PAY dynamics because the program had been stationed in a community center across town. He had seen to it that program staff produced monthly reports for the City Life Institute and provided detailed case management records of their clientele for routine organizational audits. However, the administrator said he had heard rumors that the program was not running at full speed at the end of the demonstration period.

The administrator outlined the story of the first evaluation firm. The firm had been selected through a routine competitive process. As the PAY program was being organized, the City Life Institute had mailed requests for proposals (RFPs) to most of the area's program evaluators. A committee comprised of staff from PAY and the City Life Institute then reviewed the submitted proposals.

The firm that was selected through the review process had designed an experimental model for its evaluation work. An experimental model compares pretests and posttests of groups who are assumed to be affected by the program with pretests and posttests of groups in a comparison situation who are assumed to be unaffected by the program. As part of the experimental model, half of the youths who were preparing for discharge from the residential treatment centers were randomly assigned to participate in PAY, and the remaining youths were assigned to participate in a control group, which used the conventional aftercare programs (with case management/counseling only). Clients from both groups would be given pretest surveys early in the first year and posttest surveys at the end of the three-year grant period. Staff from both programs would also conduct routine assessments and maintain case management records on each client. The evaluation firm then planned to analyze the pre- and posttest data, and compare any changes in youth behavior in the conventional aftercare program to changes in youth behavior in the PAY program. The case management records would be used for additional analysis and to help interpret findings, where relevant.

However, three issues affected the evaluation process. First, program staff had been instrumental in selecting the evaluation firm, but they had no formal training in evaluation methodology. They may not have understood that random selection was key to the utility of this evaluation design. When the evaluation firm gave them a list of youths being discharged from the residential treatment centers, with half assigned to PAY and half assigned to the conventional aftercare program, staff balked. The staff wanted some choice in hand-selecting their clientele (which could also skew evaluation results in favor of the PAY program). They ended up selecting their clients from the Opportunities Fair they organized for residential treatment clients early in the program's first year. Purportedly, staff referred 120 youths to PAY from the fair but never notified the evaluation firm of the change in protocol. Most of the remaining participants in the fair were slated to participate in conventional aftercare programs.

Second, the evaluation staff did not conduct their own pretest and posttest surveys. Instead they assigned this duty to staff from the program and control group, possibly for budgetary reasons. Moreover, for unknown reasons the evaluation firm never requested the pretest surveys at the time they should have been conducted.

Third, the evaluation team assumed an external posture to the program. Evaluators who select the external stance often limit their involvement in the program to planning an evaluation design, developing questionnaires and other measurement instruments, and conducting pretest surveys (or at minimum monitoring others who conduct the surveys)—then tend to back away from the program until it is time to conduct posttests. This external stance was almost a standard in the field until the late 1970s, when evaluation reformers and funding agencies began to recognize the value of using evaluation feedback to improve programs in progress (e.g., Patton, 1978).

The PAY evaluation team maintained minimal contact with program personnel from early in the first year to late in the program's third year. At this time the evaluation firm began contacting PAY staff to request the pretest and posttest surveys from clients. The evaluators received no response from staff despite repeated (and documented) contacts by telephone, fax, and mail. Finally, just as the program was about to close, the evaluation firm received a box of seventy-five files of PAY case management records, with a short note from staff informing the evaluation team that no one had conducted pretest or posttest surveys, or maintained the random sample the evaluators had drawn for clientele. At this point, the evaluation firm notified the parent organization that the terms of their contract had not been kept and they could not proceed with the evaluation.

When asked if our consulting firm could conduct an evaluation at this late date, I told them it was possible, but it would involve clearcut design limitations. I said our evaluation team probably could access enough client names and telephone numbers from PAY's case management records and from the records of the conventional aftercare programs to conduct telephone interviews. Our team would employ a quasi-experimental evaluation design in which we would construct a comparison group by selecting youth from the conventional aftercare programs that matched the PAY youths in certain salient characteristics (e.g., age, race/ethnicity, type of residential treatment center client utilized), but who reported receiving no PAY services. Using the original pre- and posttest instrument as a model, we could pose questions retrospectively, asking clients about their current situation at the close of a three-year program and their situation three years ago as they entered the program.* We also acknowledged that our results might be affected by the staff decision to handpick their clients (potentially skewing findings in favor of the program), and we would be addressing this limitation in our report. As we do routinely, we strengthened the overall design with analyses of additional data sources, including qualitative interviews with program stakeholders (e.g., client parents, staff from collaborating organizations) and program documents (e.g., the case management records, program reports). Our team received the go-ahead from the City Life Institute.

---

*Retrospective pretesting has been shown to be an effective strategy in several studies (Howard, 1980; Aiken & West, 1990).

The administrator was able to locate only one of PAY's former staff members to help guide our effort. The available man, "Mark," was currently employed in another City Life effort, and at first seemed quite willing to help us with all of our needs. He transported the box of seventy-five case management records from the first evaluation firm to us, expressing surprise that his files were not included in the box. He said he would search for his own records and get back to us. He also gave us some unsettling information. He said that PAY's staff supervisor had been unable to control his staff. Following the initial flurry of activity planning the Opportunities Fair, some staff began coming to work "when they felt like it." According to Mark,

> He [staff supervisor] even started a sign-in/sign-out sheet at the desk so people would have to tell him where they were going. They'd walk right by the sheet and just say they had to be out in the field today. [Name] would just come in to pick up his check every other Friday. You'd never see him any other time.

However, the case management files in the box appeared to provide more than enough information to begin the process of accessing PAY clients. In addition to names, telephone numbers, addresses, and signed parental permission slips for the program and evaluation, each client's file also included weekly progress reports, assessments, lists of activities accomplished, and a substantial number of referral forms to other sources of support. The names and telephone numbers of clients were given to the evaluation interviewers to conduct the telephone surveys (with the hope that Mark would soon deliver his records as well). I began coding the files for descriptive data and contacting individuals at the referral sources to schedule qualitative interviews. I also read the PAY reports on program activities and services, including the semiannual reports to the federal funding agency and the monthly reports to the parent organization. These appeared to be potential sources of descriptive data for the evaluation.

Our original optimism quickly waned. The data from the reports lacked the details that would have been useful for an evaluation report, even though the information suggested that PAY had been meeting its goals and timelines. This was not the case with the other data sources. I personally began conducting the qualitative interviews with stakeholders. The results were consistent. Personnel from the conventional aftercare programs and the purported resource programs for PAY clients (e.g., the job training and placement projects, the recreational options, the special interest clubs, and the volunteer sites) all claimed they had no contact with PAY staff after the program's first six months and had no reason to believe PAY was servicing any clients at all after that date.

We continued to request the missing client files from Mark. After claiming that his case management files were missing due to some kind of "sabotage" by other PAY staff members, we asked him to simply provide a list of his clients. He said he had the list and repeatedly promised to deliver it. We also asked him for the names of the resource sites where he said he had sent his clients. During the course of our six-month contractual period, we never received a single name from Mark.

The interviewers were also experiencing irregularities. Although they had no trouble accessing clients whose names had been provided by the conventional aftercare programs, they could locate none of the PAY clients. They reported that the telephone numbers of these youths (listed in their case management files) were either disconnected or now belonged to other parties. One interviewer told me that she tried to contact a client at a number listed in the box of files, but the party she reached claimed ownership of that number for over twenty years and knew of no way that the client could have claimed that telephone number.

I was also discovering curious entries in the case management files. While scanning these files to code for client progress indicators, I sometimes found female clients being referred to as "he" in the weekly progress reports, or male clients referred to as "she." I also noticed similar referral patterns for many clients. For example, nearly thirty job placement referrals were reported to a particular restaurant. But this restaurant was owned by one of the individuals I interviewed who claimed to have no contact at any time with PAY staff or clients. Within days I unearthed the pattern behind these incongruities. I discovered that the logs were a series of duplications. Each of the seventy-five case management files followed one of seven models. Apparently staff had created seven versions of possible files and then photocopied them, changing only the names of the clients on the cover sheet and the parental permission slips (sometimes forgetting to check for gender references in the text).

To verify that the client names were actually fraudulent, the interviewers and I visited a random sample of addresses listed for the clients. Of the fifteen we visited, eleven addresses did not exist at all. The remaining four addresses were either businesses or were occupied by individuals who claimed the "clients" could have never lived at the residences.

We were eventually able to interview a few youths who had actually received some PAY services. We did this by accessing sign-in sheets from the PAY Opportunities Fair. Over forty clients from this source did report receiving "a week or two" worth of services during the first year, but claimed no contact with staff after that. Several described the promises they had received from staff, their disappointment in trying unsuccessfully to reach staff to fulfill these referral and service promises, and their frustration in not knowing who to contact to complain about all of this.

These findings appeared in our evaluation report. The parent agency did not dispute the results and sent the report to the federal funding agency. Staff from the City Life Institute later told me they never heard from the federal funding agency after sending them the evaluation report. Nearly $1 million had been spent for a program that existed, for all practical purposes, only in a box.

In the case of the PAY project, staff created an illusion of a program with measurably fraudulent records. However, most paper program staff create illusions on a more abstract level. Some are adept at maintaining program commitments at the conceptual and processual levels for extended periods of time. Read on for the Program on the Plains example.

THE PROGRAMS ON THE PLAINS INITIATIVE: THE PLANS TO PLAN

I served on various conference committees with the man who would eventually become the coordinator of the "Programs on the Plains" initiative. He telephoned me shortly after accepting the position for the new project, stating that he needed consulting services in evaluation and research. He explained that a recently deceased resident in the Great Plains area had bequeathed $9 million to the local university and had specified that the funds were to be used to improve the (broadly defined) "health" of the farming community, but in measurable ways. Some of the funds had already been allocated to the university to conduct a local needs assessment on health-related issues. Although not a local resident himself, my acquaintance had been hired by the university to coordinate the effort under a group of faculty members. His job was to plan and implement health programming activities through area grassroots organizations.

The coordinator was not specific about his consultant needs. He arranged to have me visit his rural sites and requested literature reviews of studies on rural issues. He also spent several hours per week telephoning me about his personal dealings with the university faculty (we never billed for these hours because I perceived he was discussing the matters with me on a friendship basis). He also hired another consultant firm that basically duplicated these efforts. I felt confused over my professional relationship with the coordinator. During the first year, I was unsuccessful in reaching a contractual agreement on what the coordinator actually expected us to do, despite repeated attempts.

The coordinator periodically designed program models and flow charts of his vision for the future of the program and gave presentations on them at university meetings and national conferences. He also sent them to both consultant firms for feedback. We reviewed the models and applauded their strengths, but consistently made the same recommendations: that he should be involving the grassroots organizations in the planning process from the onset (per his clearly stated job description), and that the models—which were highly abstract and theoretical—would eventually have to include specific, measurable program services and activities. His response was that he would soon hire community developers to maintain direct contact with the grassroots groups, and he would conduct his own community needs assessment to make decisions about specific services (arguing that the needs assessment previously and recently conducted by the university was inadequate).

Year one ended. No community plan and no community programs were in place. In his reapplication proposal to the funding source, the coordinator summarized one of his models, which diagrammed program attributes for the following year. The model included components he thought he would eventually implement (e.g., nutrition, prevention of substance abuse and domestic violence) and early processes he hoped to add (e.g., community diagnosis, strategic planning).

The coordinator also called me and explained that the funding source required him to have an evaluation plan in place and he now needed to summarize one for the upcoming year. He asked me to review what he had written. He had been reading articles on empowerment evaluation (an approach that attempts to empower program staff through training in self-evaluation), and decided to use this approach for his project. In his report, he wrote that our firm was consulting with the program to train program staff in self-evaluation. He also cited an article we had published on training grassroots groups in empowerment evaluation (Lackey, Moberg, & Balistrieri, 1997). However, for some time I had been feeling an ethical conflict about continued involvement in the project and worried that the use of our name might give the appearance that actual evaluation activity had been going on—as opposed to plans for evaluation activity. I told the coordinator that I had mixed feelings about the empowerment evaluation approach and that my article (which he apparently had not actually read) pointed out more shortcomings than benefits in this self-assessment approach. I also suggested that he read other critiques on the approach and gave him specific citations. He responded that he did not want to give up control over the evaluation process—hence this was why he made the decision to go with the self-evaluation approach. We ended the conversation with a compromise. He deleted any use of our firm's name that could suggest that we were making decisions on evaluation approaches or methodologies and the reference to my article (that he had previously cited as supportive of the empowerment approach). We would continue to advise the program on research issues, when asked.

Year two ended. During this year, I had less contact with the program. As had been planned, the coordinator hired two community developers. Their roles were to attend a limited number of grassroots meetings and interview community residents about their needs. They tape-recorded interviews using essentially the same questionnaire designed by the researchers who conducted the first needs assessment. They also conducted surveys. The coordinator occasionally telephoned me to discuss the progress on the needs assessment and departmental dynamics—particularly his concerns that one member of the university faculty was beginning to question the lack of progress in implementing program activities. The coordinator said he had told the faculty member that the needs assessment was still in progress, and the completed plan would emerge from these findings. He also told me that the community developers had now conducted nearly 100 interviews with over 1,000 pages of transcripts, and announced that he was "not going to read all that." I then suggested that we read and analyze these data (including the surveys) and produce a report. This could help the initiative while finally giving us an opportunity to negotiate a contract for specific services.

The coordinator accepted this suggestion and said he would go immediately to the disgruntled faculty member and explain that the report was now in progress. He said the faculty member might be placated if delivered an actual product.

Early in the third year of the project, our firm analyzed the data. In over 1,000 pages of transcripts, we were able to learn a great deal about the needs of the rural community. One point we also learned was that those interviewed had no idea what Programs on the Plains was supposed to be doing for them. Throughout the interviews, they posed questions about the project to the community developers, who in turn gave inexplicit responses (perhaps because they were not clear themselves about what the project was funded to do or perhaps because they were instructed to be inexplicit). From these data, we produced a reader-friendly report of approximately 100 pages, including both the survey and interview results. At the close of the report, we summarized all findings and presented a series of recommendations on very specific service needs, based on the findings. The day the coordinator received the report, he telephoned me, stating that he was quite pleased with the report overall, but he asked me to delete the recommendations at the end. "If the community people read this," he argued, "they will expect us to actually provide these services for them, not realizing that these are *your* recommendations." I said I understood and deleted the section. He then said that he had decided to hold a Programs on the Plains conference for community residents, and project staff could at last begin the planning process through resident connections made there.

As soon as the needs assessment was finalized, I ended my working relationship with the project, citing philosophical and other differences. Just over a year later I telephoned the coordinator on an unrelated issue. Following our conversation, I asked him how the project was going. He said that the needs assessment had been very successful and that over 500 reports had been given out thus far. I questioned him about other activities and he said, "Things were still in the planning stages." I asked about the proposed conference and he told me they were "still expecting to do something along that line— perhaps not that specifically."

Thus despite two published needs assessments, an ongoing series of program models, and continuous reports that summarized "plans to plan," the Programs on the Plains initiative was years old and had apparently produced no final plan or actual services for the local residents—none at least beyond the processes that resulted in paper products. Again, close to $1 million had been spent on paper products only. How can this happen?

THE STORIES BEHIND THE STORIES

Neither PAY nor Programs on the Plains produced the services they were funded to provide. But both programs continued with no apparent repercussions. During this time, the programs' funding remained intact, staff held their positions, potential consumers of service staged no public outcry, and the media never exposed the lack of program performance. Again, how can this happen? A number of factors were operating simultaneously. Two factors were the growing global acceptance of representation as reality and the lack of accountability mechanisms in the social service industry.

Representation As Reality

Staff from the two programs lived in a wider world in which the representation of the real was quickly supplanting the real. People rarely questioned whether the images they received appropriately portrayed concrete human interaction. In everyday life, TV images had become our community news, businesses were assessed by printed annual reports and projections rather than actual business transactions, audiences of TV evangelists became our faith communities, paper reports of "prepaid forward contracts" hid corporate debt, and Internet chat rooms were hailed as "town hall meetings." Virtual reality, or simulacra, was becoming habitus. The virtual was no longer an alternative to real phenomena, but had in many cases replaced it. Baudrillard (1994) summarized this substitution process:

> It is no longer a question of imitation, nor duplication, nor even parody. It is a question of substituting the signs of the real for the real, that is to say of an operation of deterring every real process via its operational double, a programmatic, metastable, perfectly descriptive machine that offers all the signs of the real and short-circuits all its vicissitudes. (p. 2)

The staff of PAY and Program on the Plains lived in this changing environment. They worked in a system where the representations of programs became the proof that these programs existed. Progress reports, in most cases, had replaced on-site monitoring. The staff were professionals with social service education and training, and years of experience in human service organizations. They had skills in creating carefully crafted proposals and reapplications, building program images through computer-generated flowcharts and conceptual models, designing public relations documents, creating program Web pages, giving formal presentations (even through digital media), and producing timely reports to monitoring agencies. They left paper trails sufficient to satisfy parent organizations, funding agencies, and—in the case of PAY—even organizational audits. In actuality, their programs delivered almost none of the activities or services their grants stipulated.

Lack of Accountability Mechanisms

Other factors fed into the practice of representation as reality. In the social service delivery system, there are four ostensible sources of accountability for programs:

1. The potential service consumers (e.g., clientele, general public)
2. The funding sources
3. Program evaluators
4. The program's sponsoring or parent organizations

All of these are affected by their relative positions in the system, as discussed next.

Service Consumers As Monitors

Of all the accountability sources, the potential consumer of services (i.e., the client, the general public) exercises the least amount of power over social programs. Consumer control is continually constrained by third-party payment and the concept of "professional expertise" (Derber, Schwartz, & Magrass, 1990; Friedson, 1984; Kirschner, 1986). Because the system elevates the judgment of the educated health or human service professional over that of the consumer, those eligible to receive services are often in the unhappy position of having to accept anything they receive or, for that matter, accept what they are denied. In addition, most of the services that consumers are eligible to receive are paid for through insurance agencies or third-party grants. These funding sources routinely limit competition, arguing that competition in this domain is tantamount to duplication of services. This leaves consumers with little say in the quality of services they can access. In the for-profit sector, consumers have at least some control in the marketplace. A McDonald's would not stay in operation long if its consumers routinely received a fraction of the orders they purchased. A plumber would end up with few repeat customers if he or she produced only paper trails of the work that had been requisitioned. A corporate department head would be sent back to the drawing board if he or she tried to explain productivity with flow charts of unmeasurable components. Any of these organizations would soon be put out of business if their employees showed up for work at will.

Human service consumers in the United States have not been completely powerless. For example, mental health communities through organizations such as the Alliance of the Mentally Ill (AMI) have been successful in organizing for improved and increased services. The Welfare Rights Organization once had representatives at most major AFDC (Aid to Families with Dependent Children) sites in the country, advising recipients on the services they could access, efficacious complaint and appeal procedures, and organized movements consumers could join to ensure continued delivery of services. But groups such as these are anomalies, and for good reasons.

First, it is very difficult for groups to organize to ensure services when the general public does not even know what these services are. Members of the general public have little knowledge of what social service options exist in their communities, much less who they serve. There are rarely any forms of Yellow Pages for social programs. Even if there were such publications, social programs change so quickly in response to the funding and political environments that any Yellow Pages edition would be obsolete in a matter of weeks. Second, even when consumers are able to learn about programs through word-of-mouth or referrals, they may never succeed in accessing the services and activities the programs are funded to provide. A potential consumer may read a brochure stating that the "Acme Program" offers family counseling, and the potential consumer may then telephone the program to receive counseling. If no one ever returns the call, the potential consumer is out in the cold. Rarely will any consumer know the name of the parent agency (if one exists) or the funding source, and even if this were known, there probably would be no procedures in actual practice at either place to appropriately process the complaint. (Chapter 4, "The Paper Information Lines," describes in more detail the influence of the media on what the public knows about these programs.)

Funding Sources As Monitors

The general public may view a program funding source as its ultimate monitor, but in actuality, private foundations and government funding agencies are motivated by many of the same needs as the social service organizations. Personnel keep their positions by demonstrating they supported or recommended the right efforts. Fund developers for these foundations or public agencies must show that the programs their institutions sponsor are serving the public well. Representation as reality is again key. At times it is difficult to distinguish the program representations filtered through funding sources from those filtered through the social service organizations. Anyone visiting a local foundation will quickly notice the number of full-color brochures and booklets in the reception areas—all portraying their grantees delivering an abundant selection of services to enrich the community.

Most evaluators deal routinely with the public funding sources. Several times a year, a program evaluator can expect a call from an officer of a governmental funding agency, asking for any anecdotal or statistical information that this officer can use to demonstrate some program success. Public funding agencies must constantly justify their programs (and actually their existence) to lawmaking bodies through some optimistic representations of the initiatives they support.

Also unlike the common public perception, funding sources rarely monitor social programs closely. Of the fifty-five programs for which we served as evaluation or research consultants, fifty-two of them were funded externally. Of these, I can recall only three instances in which the funding agency maintained hands-on contact with the program (and this usually amounted to a telephone call once a month to the program's director—not contact with the program clients). All of the other funding sources required no more than some form of periodic written report and at times staff attendance at meetings or conferences (rarely more than biannually). Site visits were rare and, when they occurred at all, never occurred more than once a year.

In fact, some personnel from funding agencies were almost inaccessible. We evaluated a program in which a new director had been hired to manage a program undergoing internal dissent. The director hoped to involve the grant officer from a public funding source in facilitating a solution. The director tried in vain to reach the officer, explaining her dilemma daily through messages on the telephone and by e-mail. After a month with no response, the director gave up. The program operated for another year and a half until the grant ended. During this time, the director never heard from the officer.

Getting private foundations to act is often equally problematic. Several years ago, we were placed under contract to evaluate a program in an eastern state. The program was funded to set up an information center to help urban families access resources. Under the terms of our contract, the program would supply us with a list of these center clients and we would conduct telephone pre- and posttest interviews. For nearly a year we requested the list and no one returned our messages. Finally the program director called and simply told us that the program had been unsuccessful in drawing families into the center (i.e., there were no clients). Several weeks after we ended our relationship with the program, we received a form letter from the funding source (a national foundation) asking us if we had submitted an evaluation report. I wrote back explaining that there was no evaluation because there was no program. One of the foundation's grant officers then mailed us a short letter stating that she would pass on my letter to the staff of the program. Within six months, we received an annual report from the national foundation. The report highlighted this particular program, the services it was funded to provide, and the information center that had been developed. In the article were full-color photographs of the program staff (but no clients) at the center.

Program Evaluators As Monitors

The general public may also view the professional evaluator as an efficacious monitor of program activities, particularly if the evaluator is not an employee of the organization being evaluated. The label of "objective outsider" is often attributed to this role. But two issues must be considered.

First, external evaluators more often than not have their own conflicts of interest. Most independent research consultants and consultant firms (like ours) rely heavily on evaluation contracts that are funded through the program that is to be evaluated. It is not known what proportion of evaluations overall are funded in this manner, particularly among the institutionally based evaluation firms. However, the director of the university evaluation center where I spent years of employment estimates that during the center's history approximately 70 percent of their contracts had also been financed this way. How are these decisions made? The ultimate funding source of the social program will usually stipulate in the RFP that an evaluation must be conducted, the proportion of the program's budget that should go for evaluation, and who will select the evaluator. In the overwhelming majority of these cases, the organization being funded is asked to select its own evaluator. Some of these organizations will then initiate a competitive process in which they issue RFPs to a number of eligible candidates. But in my experience, few of those who review the evaluation proposals actually have any training in evaluation. Most of the time it is the staff of the program or the sponsoring organization that are responsible for the reviews. In other cases, no competitive processes exist. Program staff are simply free to select anyone they wish to conduct the evaluation. These contracts are then usually offered on an annually renewable basis. According to Weiss (1998),

> It even happens that an outside research firm will try to sweeten the interpretation of program results (by choice of respondents, by selection of data) in order to ingratiate itself with the agency managers and be first in line for further contracts. (p. 38)

Second, trendy new evaluation approaches increasingly have divested the evaluator of autonomy. During the days of the Great Society, some early evaluators abused their roles when they were more intent on pursuing their own interests and impressing their scientific peers than on satisfying the needs of clients or the interests of stakeholder groups (Shadish, Cook, & Leviton, 1991). In response to those abuses, many (including myself) welcomed the more democratic approaches to research and evaluation that followed, including participatory action research (Tax, 1958; Whyte, 1991), utilization-focused evaluation (Patton, 1997), interpretive/constructivist evaluation (Guba & Lincoln, 1989), democratic evaluation (House, 2003), and collaborative/participatory evaluation (Cousins & Earl, 1995). All of these approaches advocated for the involvement of key stakeholder groups in developing the research plans, including program personnel, volunteers, administrators, collaborators, and consumers of services.

However, a recent genre called *empowerment evaluation* has taken this movement in quite another direction. Fetterman (1994) proposed an approach whereby evaluators train key stakeholders to conduct their own evaluations and learn techniques to advocate for their program (Fetterman also suggested that professional evaluators play roles in the advocacy process). When originally proposed, empowerment evaluation could have also included consumers of services among those empowered to self-evaluate, but as this genre was refined in practice, references to consumers were dropped and only program staff received training in the self-evaluations (Fetterman, 1996; Scriven, 1997). Scriven (1997), suggesting that this movement had already become an international one, described the consequences:

> After all, empowerment evaluation, as Fetterman most recently defines it . . . means having a program evaluate its own performance—and whatever you call it, that is hardly the state of the art in controlling bias. . . . It is a larger further step to give the evaluees veto power over the evaluation design or operation, and a yet further one to suggest that the staff should design and implement the evaluation. . . . The arguments for these extensions are very appealing to staff, and very dangerous for consumers. (pp. 169-170)

For more on the role of the evaluator in monitoring programs, see Chapter 6.

Parent Organizations As Monitors

The general public may regard the sponsoring or parent organizations as legitimate monitors of the programs they offer. In some cases they are. Directors of community centers, for example, usually have ongoing contact with the general public. Because of the nature of programming, consumers of services are often together in large numbers. Consumers can share experiences with each other and give instant feedback to program staff and organizational leaders. But in most cases, chains of command or layers of bureaucracy separate agency leaders from the general public.

Perrow (1972) also made the case that the point of reference for most organizations is the system, not the general public. In his watershed work on complex organizations, the author argued that organizations should not be viewed as responding to the environment, but rather as shaping the environment, culture, and society. He critiqued functionalist ideas that portray organizations as collectively carrying out the public good. Although Perrow contended that organizations are necessary structures within postindustrial societies, he also depicted them as imperfect tools under the control of imperfect "masters." According to the author, "The major aspect of the environment of organizations is other organizations: the citizen and the community fall between the stools" (p. 203).

Along the same line, Meyer and Rowan (1977) identified "myths and ceremonies" that organizations employ to legitimate their activities. Certain expected (institutionalized) organizational practices carry competitive advantages—practices that are viewed as evidence of organizational effectiveness and merit. Thus organizations present images to the outside world that signal their compliance with institutionalized expectations—even though these external representations may be decoupled from day-to-day internal operational reality. These portrayals to the outside world replace real accountability in institutionalized organizations, while at the same time increasing the viability of the organizations.

Some of the practices that serve as status markers within the social service delivery system are represented as if they were accountability linkages to the general public. Two examples are program evaluations and needs assessments. An organizational leader may publicly announce that the organization is about to commission an evaluation of a particular program or is planning a study to assess community needs. Researchers may then conduct surveys with program clients or door-to-door interviews with residents to assess needs, and the impression conveyed is that the organization is doing all it can to be accountable to the will of program consumers and the general public. But in reality, needs assessments and evaluation reports (even the positive ones) are only occasionally distributed beyond organizational walls, and report findings are seldom used in organizational planning.

The largest community assessment I ever led was commissioned by a public agency to determine neighborhood development needs in an urban area. Over twenty researchers worked on the study, which included nearly 600 resident interviews and over 3,000 windshield surveys (checkoff forms for commercial and residential properties) of neighborhood assets. Ostensibly the study was to be used to guide planning processes for a major development project the agency was about to initiate. Several years after submitting the 150-page report on our findings, I was introduced to the individual who had become the development project's director. The project was then near completion. After the introduction she said, "I've heard your name somewhere before." I told her I was the lead researcher on the needs assessment for her project. She then replied, "Oh, yes, I'd heard there'd been some kind of a study." Another paper product remained just that.

AND THE STORY DOES NOT END HERE

Hence, what has increasingly occurred in the social service delivery system is the advancement of a cultural practice by which the representation of a program can supplant the actual program. In addition, the potential mainstays of accountability—the service consumers, funding sources, program evaluators, and sponsoring agencies—have either been steadily divested of power or are co-opted within this system. But there is more to the story. There is another form of human service initiative in which accountability dissipates even further. This is the social program in the form of a community-wide coalition. Read on.

Chapter 3

The Paper Coalitions

Chapter 2 discussed lack of accountability mechanisms in individual social service programs. In those cases, service consumers can at least identify a chain of command in the programs. But when entire coalitions* of organizations are responsible for coordinating or implementing programs, they are further removed from sources of accountability.

The three examples of coalitions presented in this chapter are taken from initiatives I evaluated in cooperation with other evaluation partners—in two cases a local university, and in another case a second evaluation firm. In all three cases, I acted as lead evaluator.

REDUCE: THE STRATIFIED COALITION

"REDUCE," which stood for Reducing and Eradicating Drug Use through Coalition Efforts, was a federally funded, five-year project designed to build the infrastructure for a coalition of organizations and coordinate and implement actual programs for the prevention of illegal drug use. The project was somewhat problematic from the start, as the funding source had ambiguous requirements about the kinds of programming and coordinating mechanisms the coalition was supposed to implement, but had very clear goals on outcomes—the coalition was supposed to reduce illegal drug use in measurable and significant ways in their region. The federal grant was awarded to a lead organization with the charge of forming the coalition across the

---

*There are different kinds of coalitions (e.g., policy-changing coalitions, advocacy coalitions), but the coalitions that this chapter addresses are networks of organizations and groups designed to plan and provide social or human service programs.

doi:10.1300/5556_03   25

rural-urban divide in a southeastern state. However, the lead organization was itself a major funding agency in the region; thus the organizational members it brought into the collaboration were compromised from the start.

The project began when the administrators of the lead organization called upon several organizations they were already funding to form the coalition and write a proposal to a federal center to support the coalition. Invited to the table were directors of major drug use prevention organizations and heads of medical centers. Joining them were government leaders, business leaders, university faculty, and informal (i.e., volunteer) community leaders. Personnel from the lead organization wrote the proposal and the coalition's grant received funding.

Three separate levels of REDUCE activity evolved in the project. The first was the lead organization and the formal coalition its administrators had formed. The role of the formal coalition was to set policy for REDUCE at all levels. Personnel from the lead organization spent a great deal of time each month preparing lengthy paper reports to the formal coalition. At no time did I ever see a packet of less than forty color-coded pages of information given to coalition members. For over a week before each coalition meeting, the lead organization's staff planned for the meetings—collecting national and local statistics, requesting information from other organizations, and reproducing publications to fill these packets. The information only occasionally related to actual REDUCE activities. Most of the reports centered on information gathered on drug use, copies of articles on prevention theories, and organization promotional material. Discussions at coalition meetings centered on program models, drug use prevention theories, and issues of coalition infrastructure (such as debates over names and charges of committees). When votes on policy were on the table, in nearly every case we observed, the formal coalition voted to support the recommendations of the lead organization. Few of the informal community leaders stayed on as permanent members of the coalition, as the meetings were routinely scheduled during workdays when the informal community leaders were at their family-supporting jobs.

Beneath this level were two subgroups—committees and an outreach component. The main committee, the Prevention Coordination Committee, worked on a major stated goal of the project (per the original proposal), which was the development of a permanent structure to coordinate drug use prevention services in the region. This structure would ideally reduce service duplications and fill service gaps with new programs. During the first year, this committee of service providers presented a plan to develop this structure. However, the lead organization's administrators expressed dissatisfaction with the plan and refused to implement it. The formal coalition supported the lead organization on the decision. The reasons given publicly for rejecting the plan were minor, but when the committee worked to correct the minor points, the plan continued to be rejected. Members of the committee remained engaged in the same processes for nearly three years, and their efforts were routinely diffused or overruled by the lead organization, and subsequently by the coalition. (Although I was the lead evaluator for most of the five years, I was never privy to any private reasons administrators from the lead organization may have had for rejecting every draft of the plan.)

In addition to committees, the lead organization worked with some of the ethnic and community-based organizations it routinely funded to develop a separate and unlinked coalition of six outreach workers. The role of these outreach workers was ostensibly to gather information from grassroots groups and advise the coalition, its committees, and the lead organization on issues affecting these specific target populations. For the full five years, the consultants met weekly with each other and one other coalition staff member to discuss information they had gathered on issues considered to be important in their target communities. These staff had no scheduled meetings with the administrators of the lead organization, nor did they have any official reporting function to the coalition. (The coalition staff member did have ongoing contact with the lead organization's administrators, but expressed frustration to the evaluators that her suggestions were rarely acted upon.) The outreach workers and the organizations they represented were also given no power at all to implement plans, programs, or services. Some of the outreach workers helped their target communities with process issues, such as meeting planning or assessing needs, but these activities were performed on a mostly discretionary basis.

For nearly the entire grant period, the committees met and outreach workers met. Conversations at these meetings did not resemble conversations at the formal coalition level. The outreach workers reiterated the concerns expressed by their target communities about growing drug dealing and drug houses. The Prevention Coordination Committee met and discussed members' tallies of prevention service gaps and duplications. Some member of the evaluation team attended nearly every coalition, committee, and outreach meeting. Not once over the years did our group hear mention of the words "drug dealing" or "drug houses," and only once was the subject of service duplications or gaps introduced at the coalition meetings, and that was in response to a proposal by the Prevention Coordination Committee (which was subsequently rejected).

Each year, some members of the evaluation team conducted an interim evaluation of the REDUCE coalition. Because no programs of any kind had been implemented in the first three years of the grant, we did not conduct any community impact surveys until the final year. However, during qualitative interviews of all who were involved in REDUCE, nearly every person complained about the control of information and the general dominance of the lead organization and how they felt constrained in being able to correct problems because their organizations were dependent on the lead organization for much of their ongoing funding.* Most of the committee members were staff at prevention organizations the lead organization funded. Nearly all of the outreach staff worked for organizations funded at least in part by the lead organization.

The evaluation reports pointed out the problems with REDUCE— the lack of efficacious linkages between the committees, the outreach efforts, and the coalition; plus the obvious failure of REDUCE to implement the efforts spelled out in the grant proposal. However, the very people who were responsible for constraining the project never actually read the evaluations (at least not those issued when I was the lead evaluator). By their own admission, the administrators of the lead organization only looked through the reports to find places where their agency's name was mentioned, and read those parts, often requesting edits to soften any negative language tied somehow to their name. (During one year, these administrators never even noticed when ten pages were duplicated by accident in the draft of the evaluation report.) Although summaries of major evaluation findings were given to coalition members, no discussion of the results or action plan to

---

*Readers may think that the practice of one funding agency giving funds to another funding agency to implement programs or coalitions might be a misguided anomaly, but we have actually seen this happen quite regularly.

address shortcomings ever resulted for the first two and one-half years. We never found any reason to believe that the federal funding agency read the evaluation reports, although copies were always sent to the agency. Grant officers came for two site visits and indicated a favorable impression of the coalition meetings they observed and the amount of paper information dispersed at the meetings (the paper products were specifically mentioned in one oral report).

No activity began on prevention programming of any kind until the fourth year of REDUCE. Late in year three, and at the continual urging of the evaluators and two of the organizations with outreach staff, the lead organization sponsored a workshop to reorganize the coalition. Most of those who participated were coalition staff, leaders of the organizations with the outreach staff, and members of their target communities. At the recommendation of these groups, the coalition was reorganized so that the majority of the members were grassroots leaders or leaders of community-based organizations. With the new coalition organized, the outreach workers were now assigned to forge a network of grassroots communities and assist them with actual programming. Several months later, the lead organization took some of their unspent funds and dispersed them to the target communities to have them sponsor local health fairs and other small programs on the theme of preventing illegal drug use. The amount expended on the mini programs was under $25,000. The total amount of the federal grant over the five-year period was over $1 million.

When we finally conducted a community-wide impact survey (only in the areas where the health fairs or other similar activities took place), 90 percent of the respondents said they had never heard of the coalition called REDUCE. No significant changes in area drug use emerged from survey findings. An independent survey conducted in the same region over the same general period of time found a substantial increase in illegal drug use by teens. When the five-year funding ran out, the coalition no longer met.

In the case of REDUCE, coalition members or organizations providing staff to the project were in clearly compromised situations, as the lead organization was also one of their major funding sources before the coalition was developed and after it dissolved. For this reason (and other minor ones), these stakeholders were not well positioned to correct a flawed effort as a paper program began to develop. But read on for a case in which failure to correct a flawed effort involved a very different set of circumstances.

TEENHEALTH: THE COALITION IN THE DARK

"TeenHealth" was also a government-supported program. The project was funded as a two-year planning grant to form a coalition and develop resources to reduce health problems among adolescents (such as obesity, teen pregnancy, substance use, eating disorders, depression, and sexually transmitted diseases). TeenHealth was implemented in a southwestern state in a county that ranked second highest in the United States in indicators of unhealthy teen behaviors, according to a national study.* Planning was not the only activity required of this project. The funding agency held a cooperative agreement with the county's social service department, which was also the coalition's lead organization, and mandated the development of an infrastructure for health promotion and prevention programming during the two-year period. The infrastructure requirement mandated extensive community organizing and the creation of neighborhood advocacy groups for later implementation of prevention plans that would be funded at a second stage.

For over a year after the social service department staff learned of the expectation, no coalition member—not even the coalition's co-chairs—were told of the community organizing or neighborhood advocacy group requirements. The department staff organized most meeting agendas around progress reports of a large-scale needs assessment the evaluation team was conducting. Despite their stated pledge to inform the coalition of all the funder's expectations, the department staff even failed to share the funder's site visit report with the coalition—a report that recommended speedy implementation of the infrastructure.

The subject of the infrastructure requirements seldom came up at the departmental meetings I attended. Concerns centered on political issues. Had they put anything in print that could offend their department heads? Was anything politically sensitive enough to call the attention of the county's elected representatives—and hence put their

---

*Because the names and identifiers of the programs in this book are changed, the study is not cited here.

jobs in jeopardy? Each sentence of print went through at least three levels of checks before being issued to any member of the public—particularly the coalition.

Evaluation feedback on lack of progress on the required infrastructure ended up being counterproductive. I was the lead evaluator on the project and it was my responsibility to express concerns during feedback sessions about lack of progress on the infrastructure. I did this and nothing followed. I later informed one of the coalition cochairs of the requirements. The cochair resigned from the coalition within days of my conversation with her (citing time constraints as her reason for resigning) and never shared the information I had given her with other coalition members (at least not to my knowledge). Shortly after her resignation, I was summoned to a meeting of social service department supervisors where I was reminded that I was a consultant funded through them and was told that they considered it inappropriate for me to speak to coalition members about anything. The social service department requested that I step back and assume an external role to the project. At this time I should have simply refused to do this, but I confess to feeling very intimidated (in fact stunned) by the verbal reprimand and their assumption that I was somehow beholden to them because they paid for the evaluation. Without reflection, I found myself agreeing to abide by their wishes. The two-year planning period came to an end with not even a mention of the required community organizing and neighborhood advocacy groups at coalition or committee meetings. This was a coalition thoroughly in the dark.

In our evaluation report on the two-year project, I pointed out the requirement of the community organizing and neighborhood advocacy groups, but I had difficulty making a strong case for any other problems with the project. Because the coalition members knew little about this or other requirements, they tended to speak in fairly positive terms about the planning grant effort. They spoke highly of the needs assessment we had conducted and the professionalism of meetings they attended, praising the valuable handouts and interesting speakers. The lack of effort on the required infrastructure apparently eluded the funding source as well (which had undergone staff turnover by the close of the two-year period), as they funded the project for the second stage, which was a five-year implementation grant. By this time, I had recovered my ethical stance and declined the opportunity to be considered as lead evaluator for the implementation grant. (Chapter 4 discusses some interesting developments on the implementation grant.)

These two examples demonstrate ways that coalitions can operate at a place far removed from the citizenry the funded projects are supposed to impact, replacing needed grassroots work with paper products. Read on for an example where the needs for paper products played a role in significantly diminishing a collaborative effort.

PROJECT UNITED-ARE-WE:
A COALITION UNITED IN NAME ONLY

"Project United-Are-We" was funded by a large private foundation and a government agency and was designed to bring together a large health care institution with grassroots partners. The effort began as a collaboration between a medical complex (including hospitals, clinics, and other health care facilities) and central city community centers in an East Coast city. As the medical complex was experiencing more victims of domestic and street violence in their emergency rooms, they worked with their partners, contacted local legislators, held press conferences, and were eventually able to convince an alliance of legislators and private funding agencies to fund a program that would provide resources for the victims. The goal of the coalition was to offer aftercare services to victims of violent crimes and their families. The lead organization in the partnership was a hospital in the medical complex, and the grant funds were distributed through them to other health care partners (the community centers did not receive direct funding from the coalition). The role of the health care component was to provide health and psychological services to the victims, which included direct medical services, social work, and treatment for posttraumatic stress. The health professionals would then refer the families to the community centers, and center staff had the charge of helping the victims and their families reintegrate into their communities (or in some cases new communities), get involved in support groups, and participate in diversionary leisure-time activities. My role as an evaluation consultant was to conduct a short-term process evaluation of the program's implementation.

The program proved to be overly complicated from the start. The health care facilities had complex paperwork requirements, often legally mandated because of medical and confidentiality issues. But at other times the paperwork just involved bureaucratic "passports," such as referral forms, vouchers for materials, and lengthy forms to request nonconfidential information. Because representatives of the community centers began working with the victims while they were still in the hospital, the community staff were asked to comply with many of the same paperwork requirements as the health care staff. Errors abounded. Community center personnel were more accustomed to an informal environment where transactions involved face-to-face contact and little paperwork. To address these issues, the leaders of the coalition scheduled a series of in-service training sessions. However, the sessions were set up chiefly to meet the needs of the health care bureaucracy—not the growing frustration of the community center staff. At least four of every five hours of in-service time I attended were devoted to procedural processes and rules on filling out the appropriate assessments and forms for the health care divisions. Tensions swelled on both sides.

Among the findings, the evaluation report cited an overemphasis on the needs of the medical bureaucracy and not enough attention paid to the ongoing issues faced by the community centers, particularly their frustration with meeting the needs of the health care bureaucracy and lack of funding. Shortly after the report was issued, the medical complex and the community centers radically altered their working relationships, and the hospital hired its own "community" workers, placing them inside the medical complex. The roles of these community workers were to talk to the victims and inform them of resources in their neighborhoods. What had begun as a coalition with institutional and grassroots components ended up being a program operated solely by the health care partner and implemented within the walls of the health care institution. The partnership aim still appeared in some of the project's printed materials but in practice had been reduced significantly.

THE STORIES BEHIND THE STORIES

There is no mystery why large-scale funding sources would want to fund coalitions rather than individual programs to address known needs. Human problems are usually broad-based. Problems may have their roots in the physical environment, neighborhoods, families, peer groups, biochemical makeup of individuals, schools, political policies, personality disorders, economic circumstances, business trends, international practices, and on and on. Where problems are multifaceted, solutions must be as well. Addressing broad-based problems through coalitions of organizations and other influential entities is the logical best choice.

Furthermore, the practice of awarding large grants to powerful lead organizations is also a logical best choice. Reviewers of proposals for large grants are going to be concerned that potential lead organizations have the leverage in their communities to draw the needed partners to the table and, of course, have the infrastructure necessary to manage large grants. Organizations such as funding agencies and government departments clearly have the infrastructure and, more important, the leverage. It is not the idea of using coalitions or powerful lead organizations to develop solutions that is flawed. Rather, it is the processes that take place all the way through the system—processes that end up subsuming what should be the main motivation at every level and every sitting, which is correcting the problem(s) the coalitions are set up to address.

What are some of these processes? In the three examples presented in this chapter, an obvious problem is the power the lead organization can exert, which could lead to positive results but also to negative ones. The issues here are really no different than they are for individual programs. The interests of the citizenry or consumers of services are simply not always what drives powerful and complex organizations. As was pointed out in Chapter 2, the point of reference for most complex organizations is often the system, not the general public (Perrow, 1972). Leaders in these bureaucracies advanced in their positions by understanding the need to present a relatively flawless image to others in their environment, while responding to internal demands of their organizations. For example, executives of the local funding agency leading the REDUCE coalition expressed concern that their agency's name was not directly linked to negative evaluation findings (hence, they reviewed only those parts of the evaluation reports I produced that included the agency name). Staff from the county department leading the TeenHealth coalition spent the greater part of their meetings trying to avoid political pitfalls tied to the project that would put their jobs in jeopardy. The hospital staff leading Project

United-Are-We insisted that the community center staff conform to the bureaucratic rules of their own health care organizations, even as they saw that it was jeopardizing their community partnerships.

However, something else is at work here as well. Because the coalition is needed to address problems that have roots at varying levels of society, those the lead organization invites to the table should be leaders and citizens from these varying social levels. But here we often find culture conflict. Richards (1996) described lessons learned from seven community health care partnerships that had developed across the country in the 1990s. Among the issues the author pointed out were differences in community and health care representatives' perceptions of accountability. According to the author, community representatives saw clearly "that their role is to be accountable to the people of their communities, to work to increase people's control over their lives" (p. 20). On the other hand, health care professionals continued to train in tertiary care hospitals "culturally removed from people, communities and all but the effects of community problems" (p. 13). Richards maintained that health staff working out of institutional settings viewed themselves as accountable primarily to the goals and needs of their individual departments. Although the holistic approach to public health problems was often a stated ideal, most health centers were a differentiated, segmented, loosely organized system of units, each operating almost autonomously. The author explained that community representatives, who experienced daily life holistically, usually did not understand the structural influences on many health care providers. Although Richards only studied the outcomes of coalitions attempting to forge partnerships between community groups and health care providers, the same argument could be made about partnerships between community groups and other complex organizations, such as large social service agencies. These organizations also have a differentiated, segmented, loosely organized system of semiautonomous units, where staff see themselves as accountable primarily to the goals and needs of their individual departments. The gradual development of cultural norms within these settings through dispositions and patterned practices is what Bourdieu (1977) called habitus.

Something else is involved in this culture conflict. Lead organizations are those that plan meeting agendas and protocols. In most cases these protocols meet the comfort levels of the lead organizations and their closest allies. Rarely have I evaluated a collaborative effort in which meetings were held when volunteer coalition members could regularly attend. Meetings inevitably were scheduled around the working hours of the lead organization staff. Agenda topics centered on the interests of the lead organization staff and their close allies. A good example of this occurred in the REDUCE project when the outreach workers were gathering information from their neighborhoods on growing drug house problems, yet the phrase "drug house" was never uttered in our presence at the coalition meetings. Many coalition members (particularly before the reorganization) were highly educated and highly positioned individuals in complex bureaucracies, whose interests appeared to center more on theoretical than practical levels.

But beyond these issues, the coalition as a coordinator and provider of services presents something perhaps more problematic. The coalition must expend considerable energy feeding itself. It is difficult enough to ask coalition members to take time away from their own organizational work to collaborate to solve broad-based problems. But before they even consider doing this, they must actually develop the coalition. Most university libraries stock literally scores of books on coalition-building strategies. A highly respected text includes these steps in its coalition processes (Dluhy, 1990):

- Initial meeting
- Developing organizational structure and bylaws
- Educating and orienting coalition members
- Selecting strategies and issues
- Identifying community resources
- Diagnosing the community
- Diagnosing the public policy environment
- Choosing a coalition approach
- Selecting coalition tactics
- Educating citizens
- Acquiring resources
- Conflict management
- Sharing resources
- Merging programs
- Renewing energy
- Maintaining communication

Although all these activities are useful—and most perhaps even necessary to accomplish project goals—the potential exists for the coalition's processes to become ends rather than means to improving the surrounding community or addressing problems under their charge. The REDUCE coalition was an example of this: the staff from the lead organization worked for over a week compiling information for printed handouts for regularly scheduled coalition meetings but spent far less time planning activities that would result in the intended outcomes of the project—the reduction of illegal drug problems in the region. The processes and their paper representations became the product.

Finally, and most important, the coalition—which has been further distanced from the community it is supposed to serve by layers of its own bureaucracy—is now nearly exempt from accountability. The coalition has a name of its own but has no autonomous authority (or at least not in the ideal sense of a coalition). No single entity is responsible for carrying out or failing to carry out the coalition's mission. If the coalition's funding sources find fault with the effort, the lead organizations can argue that the partners have failed to fulfill their roles. If the local press or consumer groups learn of the existence of the coalition and want to know why the problems of focus are not improving, coalition members can cite problems with the lead organizations or other coalition partners. Credit and blame can be diffused in all directions. The conundrum of accountability reigns.

BUT THE STORY DOES NOT END HERE

It is almost time to switch gears and discuss how superb efforts emerge in this vacuum of accountability—but not quite. First, it is important to shed light on the processes of how the public actually obtains information on social service programs and coalitions. It is time to ask what the public actually knows about what is working and what is not.

Chapter 4

The Paper Information Lines

Let us recap. The social service delivery system includes four sources of accountability for programs:

1. The potential service consumers
2. The funding sources
3. Program evaluators
4. The program's sponsoring or parent organizations

Chapter 5 also discusses the great importance of ethics-based program leadership. All of these sources are affected by their relative positions in the system, and all deal with intervening factors that limit their effectiveness in monitoring programs. When entire coalitions are coordinating or implementing social programs, the accountability mechanisms dissipate further. The coalitions are distanced from potential service consumers by layers of their own bureaucracy, and credit and blame can be dispersed broadly among the various coalition members, leaving no single entity indisputably accountable.

What is left? Of course there is the American media. The free press has been described as a watchdog over uses of power and uses of taxpayer dollars. But do the media monitor social service programs? The answer is rarely. Read on for some examples of what information the public was able to access through the media on some of the projects where I acted as lead evaluator.

TEENHEALTH: THE MEDIA IN THE DARK

About seven years ago, I was traveling and stopped in the county where the TeenHealth coalition was located. As I was having breakfast

doi:10.1300/5556_04

in the hotel, I picked up the local paper. My jaw dropped when I saw the front-page headline. It read: "[Name] County Tops Nation in Unhealthy Teens." Recall from the previous chapter that TeenHealth ("the coalition in the dark") was the project that had received a multi-million-dollar grant to increase the healthy practices of teens when the county was rated the second worst in the nation in indicators of unhealthy adolescents. I read on. The article summarized the statistics and then moved into an interview with the director of the county social service department—the department that served as the lead organization for the TeenHealth coalition. This director reported being alarmed by the statistics, discussed factors that might have played roles in the problem indicators (such as the lack of parental monitoring in the homes of "latchkey teens"), and claimed the need for action to address the growing problem. I read and reread the article. Nowhere did the head of the county department or the reporter mention a word about the large TeenHealth grant the department held.

I did not have my records with me but as closely as I could recall, the TeenHealth coalition would have been late in its fourth or fifth year of the second-stage implementation grant. I wondered if they had lost the grant somewhere along the line, as it seemed virtually unfathomable that the person most responsible for overseeing these funds to correct the growing problem would have failed to mention the project in some context, or that the reporter covering this subject never heard even a rumor of the coalition's existence.

I recalled a local citizen named "Ellen" who sat on the coalition during the planning phase and who had been trying to push the project into more measurable action. I looked up her telephone number and gave her a call. As soon as I told her I was in town and had just read the paper, she started laughing. "You see how bad it's gotten?" she roared. Ellen told me that the coalition was indeed still funded but that she was no longer involved. She said she had agreed to chair a committee during the implementation stage, but when she complained about lack of action in developing programs, the department staff and a few other coalition members "reorganized the infrastructure" so that her committee was phased out. "Basically they got rid of me, the trouble maker," she laughed. Ellen said she still maintained contact with some coalition members and very little measurable work had been done to date. I asked her if she intended to call the newspaper and inform the reporter that the social service department (whose director was "alarmed" by the statistics) held this grant that was supposed to be reducing the problem. Ellen sighed and said she probably would not as she had to deal with this department in other domains and did not want to be the whistle-blower.

On my way back home, I was still shaken. I wondered what I was obligated to do as a past evaluator of the project. Should I contact the reporter? I e-mailed another evaluator who had worked on the project with me during the planning stage. He said he did not know what we should do, but given that another firm currently held the evaluation contract, it would likely be their responsibility, if any moral responsibility existed at all. I was dissatisfied with that answer, realizing how intimidated I had felt by the department's supervisors when I served as lead evaluator, and wondered if the current evaluators were feeling equally intimidated. When I arrived home, I debated with myself for about a week about my moral responsibility. If I did place the call, what should I say? Should I provide any details from my evaluation work in the planning stage? Should I simply state that the county department held this grant? Was the story now too cold for follow-up? Was my evaluation colleague correct that this really was not a responsibility that belonged in our camp?

I wrote out lists weighing the options. Eventually I had to set the problem aside to take care of more pressing concerns. Then one day I simply forgot about it. Today I deeply regret this failing on my part.

REDUCE: THE MEDIA IN THE ARTIFICIAL LIGHT

Another coalition the reader will recall from Chapter 3 was REDUCE. This was the coalition designed to decrease use of illegal drugs across a rural-urban divide. The reader may remember that the coalition was funded to develop a coordination mechanism to reduce duplications in services and fill service gaps with new drug use prevention programming. Outreach staff from ethnic and neighborhood associations had been assigned to collect information on the roots of drug abuse in their communities but were not given the authority or resources to produce programs to address these needs until the end of the grant period. No coalition-driven coordination mechanism ever emerged from the million-dollar grant and no efforts were put forth on new programming until year four of the five-year funding period.

The lead organization was a major funding agency itself in the state and had its own public relations department staffed with media-savvy (and well-connected) professionals. When the lead organization learned that one of the outreach staff had been conducting focus groups with her target population on the roots of drug abuse, the executives requested their public relations department to develop a press conference on the focus group results. The information was published in the local newspapers and on local television stations. During annual evaluation interviews, the outreach staff member responsible for the focus groups expressed frustration over the media frenzy. Her comments went something like the following:

> I won't go so far as to say I was used by them, but what I did was such a small thing—[a few] focus groups conducted with and by youth. They built this up like it was such a big deal to make it look as if this project was really doing something.

During the last year of the grant—just months before we conducted our community impact survey—the public relations staff of this organization and a coalition partner developed a series of press releases on the prevention fairs and prevention information gathered by the outreach workers. One of the public relations workers showed me a file she had developed on the topics of interest of each radio station, newspaper, informational Web site, and TV station in the target areas and how she had created stories on the prevention themes that would fit into these media topical areas. The public relations staff did not simply mail the press releases to the local media. They personally visited reporters of the TV stations and newspapers in the target areas. The reader may recall that only 10 percent of the respondents in the community-wide survey claimed they had actually heard of the REDUCE coalition at the end of the five-year project. It is difficult to estimate how many would have claimed even name recognition of the coalition without the effort put out by the public relations personnel shortly before the survey was conducted.

The examples of TeenHealth and REDUCE show ways that the public can learn or fail to learn about programs and coalitions. No objective news on these projects is simply "out there" to be gathered and published. All news has sources, and these sources are rarely media professionals gathering information on programs on their own. Our firm has never evaluated a program in an area where the local media had reporters who made routine calls on members of the social service delivery system or showed up at service sites on a regular beat to check out the level of funded services provided by the programs. Organizations with the resources to create media "pegs" or stories may choose to feed or starve the media. These decisions are made based on the motivations of organizational leaders, such as the way they predict they will be perceived in the community. Although exceptions do exist, in most cases the public simply has access to the information that is released by the organizations. Read on for examples of superb program efforts and learn what mass media information the public could access on these.

THE IMMIGRANT GARDENS: THE BLIND EYE

Our firm was commissioned to evaluate a statewide urban gardens project in a southern state. The program negotiated temporary land leases with landowners in urban areas, subdivided the land into small plots for gardening, rented the spaces out to gardeners (at rates ranging from $10 to $20 a year), held free gardening classes, and provided the gardeners with access to water and gardening supplies. City governments owned most of the vacant lots that were leased for gardening, and the land leases rarely had durations of more than one year. As soon as the land was sold or slated for other development, the gardens were plowed under. This meant that each spring the program staff in all the state's urban areas had to scurry around and find alternative land sites for displaced gardeners and then prepare the new sites for gardening. There was an exception. One of the state's cities had negotiated a series of long-term leases for a large gardening area for over twenty years. At the edge of the city, located in a cove that few local urbanites ever even saw, was a square quarter mile of undeveloped land. On this land were over 200 garden plots, referred to by the program staff as the "immigrant gardens." Most of the area's gardeners were poor, rural immigrants from various countries who were able to maintain their cultural traditions and help feed their families through the garden rental opportunities.

The last of the long-term leases for this land was about to end when the statewide program made the decision to commission an outside research firm, Jill Florence Lackey & Associates, to evaluate the statewide project. (Whether the lease arrangements had any influence on their decision to evaluate, I never knew.) This project ended up with some of the finest evaluation findings we ever published. We found a program that was first of all well implemented—that provided the resources, activities, and services stated in its funding proposals and other program documents. Consistently, over time, and across all the urban sites, the urban gardeners reported significantly more positive outcomes relating to good health, maintaining heritages, money saved on food, family cohesiveness, and sociability than comparison groups of people with similar demographic backgrounds but who did not participate in the program.

During the last months of the evaluation period, I began to hear rumors from program staff that the city that hosted the immigrant gardens was considering an offer by a large development firm to create an office complex on that land. When we completed the evaluation report, one of our recommendations for the program's future was for staff to engage in an educational effort with the multicultural/multilingual gardeners to inform them of their rights to contact their political representatives and organize in collective action to retain the land for gardening, if the development project was approved. I also told staff that I was available to give presentations to the government officials on the evaluation results, should this be needed.

A year passed. A friend of mine in this city began to send me newspaper clippings and tapes of talk shows about the debate over creation of the office complex on the quarter-mile cove. No decision had been made, primarily because some residents with homes surroundings the cove organized a protest group, contacted the media, and staged a campaign with their elected representatives to maintain the cove as undeveloped land. Eleven articles in the city's major newspaper covered the battle, and not one article included even a word about the immigrant gardeners, although over 80 percent of the cove was partitioned into the vegetable gardens. One of the state's talk radio shows had a regular feature called the Week's Most Ridiculous News Story. During one week they chose the conflict between the residents living next to the cove and the city. The radio show moderators cracked jokes about the residents wanting to keep the open land so they would have a place where their "dogs could defecate" and keep a well-defined separation between themselves and the "real" city people. The moderators expressed outrage at the city for even considering bending to the residents on the issue when the office complex was needed. No one that called in indicated any knowledge of the gardeners in the cove. After listening to the segment, I sent a letter to one of the moderators informing him what really was happening in the cove, and enclosed a copy of the executive summary of the evaluation report. I never heard from the moderator, nor did I note any clarification of the issue on succeeding shows.

After waiting over a week, I called a staff member of that city's urban gardens program and asked why the media never even mentioned the gardening program on the land. The staff member sighed and explained the reality of their situation. He said that the staff had indeed attempted to educate the gardeners on their rights, and some of the gardeners had tried to organize some resistance. However, no one could overcome problems with the language and cultural differences and the fears of some gardeners who were not yet citizens that a public protest would affect their status in this country. And why couldn't the staff themselves then advocate for their program, I asked. The program staff member explained another reality in words something like the following:

> We not only have our offices situated at no expense to us in city government office buildings, but we have to rely on the city for so many other plots of land we use outside of the "immigrant gardens" for the rest of our gardeners. We just can't afford to tick off the city.

The staff member also explained that one of his co-workers had recently sent a copy of the urban gardens evaluation report to the newspaper reporter covering the story and hoped that the paper would publish news on this.

The newspaper did. Within days, a three-paragraph article appeared in the paper with the headline that the development of the cove would also mean the eviction of over 200 gardening families. The article mentioned nothing about the positive impacts the gardens had on these families or the various ethnic groups who gardened on the land. The next series of articles returned to the theme of the battle between the residents and the city. The city won and eventually the ground was broken for the new medical office complex. The gardeners were evicted without a murmur in the media. Some had gardened in the cove for twenty years.

Odd as it may seem, this story actually ended up with a satisfying outcome. The urban garden staff—some who had worked for the program for decades—knew many of these gardeners personally. Perhaps for that reason, as well as a general commitment to their program, they worked diligently to find new homes for the gardens. Using recorded testimonials of the gardeners and the evaluation report, the staff spent two years searching for new sites. Eventually a large institution in the city donated a plot of land nearly equal in size to the land they had just lost. The land ended up having better soil quality and better access to a water supply than the land of the cove.

This example, like the story of TeenHealth, discussed the ways the media failed to publish relevant information about program activities (in part because they may have lacked sources for the information). In the next example, the media did cover events relating to another fine program we evaluated. However, the coverage hardly reflected the value of the program.

PC&C: THE STEPFORD STAFF

The "PC&C" program (Preventing Crime and Corrections) was designed to divert adolescents (ages twelve to nineteen) from the criminal justice system through (1) community service assignments as alternatives to fines for minor law violations, (2) recreational programming, (3) support groups, and (4) exposure to the realities of correctional institutions. The program routinely employed rehabilitated ex-offenders as assistants to case managers. Some of the ex-offenders had felony convictions, but none for sex offenses.

At the time our firm was selected to evaluate PC&C, I already knew something about the program. PC&C had been in operation for over fifteen years and its founder had (much later) written a book about crime prevention that was based in part on the data she collected from program clients. I had read the book. In addition, one of the main newspapers in the program's home city (a city near my residence) carried articles periodically on the program. The articles focused on an ongoing battle between a leading political figure in the area and the first director, the author of the book. In her book, the author had placed much of the blame for an increase in local youth crime on the city's political and law enforcement policies—policies she believed discriminated against families living at the poverty level.

She also impugned this particular political leader. The political leader later wrote a book of his own on issues affecting the city. In the book, he described some of what he considered to be the most ill-advised programs in the city. He mentioned PC&C by name, stating that it exposed youths to ex-offenders and put youths at risk of being victimized by them. The news media (particularly radio talk shows) covered the "book battle" between the two authors, citing the accusations on both sides.

About five years later an RFP went out to most of the state's evaluation firms, and we applied. While I was waiting to hear who had been chosen to conduct the evaluation, another war of words regarding PC&C made its way into the city's press. The program's current director was interviewed on a radio show about PC&C's upcoming recreational activities. During the interview, the director mentioned some of the systemic influences on youth crime, such as poverty and lack of family programs in the city. The local political leader heard the interview and had his staff call the press. The political leader was interviewed and called the director a "criminal apologist," and he again questioned how any organization could hire ex-felons (allegedly rehabilitated or not) to serve "children." He called for legislation to end this practice (although I do not believe that any legislation proposals materialized).

This might have been the worst possible time for our firm to conduct the evaluation. In addition to the media controversy, the program's parent organization had just undergone a major change. The organization's board—on which sat this political leader—had just hired a new executive director. Everyone at Jill Florence Lackey & Associates knew that these evaluation results could be controversial. When I announced to my staff that we had been awarded the contract, I heard nothing but groans. Nearly everyone involved stated from the onset that they expected this evaluation to be a giant headache.

We began the work expecting to see a program in disarray, due in part to the negative media coverage and to the employment of people (the ex-offenders) who we thought probably lacked strong work histories. We found nothing of the sort. The program was very large and handled over 1,000 clients each year. I had sent the program director requests for information, including descriptions of program components, sites and dates of events and activities, lists of clients with telephone numbers and addresses, names of collaborators in the correctional institutions and courts, case management records, and copies of client report cards (where the program had these). My first meeting was with the program's director, program collaborators, a few youth clients, and several program middle managers. One by one they handed over boxes and files of records of everything I requested. As part of the evaluation design, we were not in a position to assign youth randomly into the program for a variety of reasons, including the fact that the program year had already begun. Conjointly we decided on a quasi-experimental model, using a series of comparison groups of youths who had gone through the juvenile justice system for various offenses but had not participated in the program. From there we set in motion a timeline, including times and places where my staff and I would observe program activities.

As with the urban gardens effort, we found a program that was well implemented—that provided the resources, activities, and services stated in its funding proposals and other program documents. I observed at the court where the staff took referrals into the program. The middle managers, together with the ex-offenders who were assisting them, met the youth charged with law violations and their families. The staff took the youths and families into rooms where they assessed each potential client for PC&C eligibility, explained the program, and introduced them to the judges. The youths were warned that if they did not participate in all the activities of the program, they would have to pay their legal fines and the law offenses would remain on their records. Activities of the program included three months to one year of community service, restitution to victims, letters of apology to the judges and the victims, support groups, Saturday morning feedback sessions, continuous school attendance, improved grades, participation in the program's sports leagues, field trips to correctional institutions, participation in a series of life skills classes ranging from grooming to dating to cooking to job interviewing, abstaining from substance use or abuse, noninvolvement in gangs, and (of course) no repeat offenses.

With overburdened courts, the pace of recruiting the clients, explaining the requirements, and working with the judges was extremely fast. I found myself having difficulty taking notes and keeping track of who was who. I recognized from my first day of observation that the staff had no chance to explain to me what was happening in each negotiation or, for that matter, even to note my presence. At times, while writing notes, I lost the group as they scurried from waiting lines to courtrooms, to judges' chambers, and to court records rooms. At the end of each court day the middle managers, making a light jest of my inability to keep up, handed over photocopies of all the day's handwritten records of assessments, notes, and recruits.

At the end of each court day, I also interviewed employees of the courts. My first series of interviews was with the judges. The general assessment of the first judge would be echoed by those that followed. The judge told me that he had worked with this program since its beginning over fifteen years ago and had worked with one specific middle manager the entire time. (I will call this manager "Rogell.") The judge praised PC&C. "I've tried to work with other programs that claim to do the same thing," the judge stated, "but it never works out." He told me that Rogell simply never forgot a youth—not their names, their special circumstances, their agreements, and their offenses. "If they show up in the system three years later, he'll remember them." The judge asked me to make note of the reactions of Rogell's assistants—the ex-offenders. "Rogell had problems as a youth. You see him today and see what a difference he makes. These guys and the kids are in awe of him." The judge claimed that PC&C was the best program he had ever worked with, irrespective of how the program appeared in the media.

Other members of my staff followed the work of the other teams of middle managers and ex-offender assistants. The reports were very similar. Their field notes provided many examples of how the middle managers drew upon the experience of the ex-offenders when youths tried to rationalize their negative behaviors. The ex-offenders often described their own similar patterns as adolescents and charted the paths that had led to their incarcerations. The teams monitored the clients very closely. If a client did not show up for a scheduled event, the manager would telephone the client's family at home. If the team received no response by phone, the parents were called at work. If the team still received no response, the team made home visits. The cajoling was routinely gentle but applied with rigorous consistency. The staff's workload was heavy every day and the hours were long. Some of the middle managers started work at 7 a.m. and continued on into the middle of the night during seasons when their sports leagues were active. Yet their schedules seldom varied. They claimed they had discovered processes that worked for them and they rarely deviated from them. We called them the "Stepford staff" (but meant in the very positive sense of consistent service).

As some members of our evaluation team conducted the observations, others conducted pre- and posttest surveys (based on self-reports) with over 800 clients and comparison youth. The PC&C clients improved significantly over the one-year pre- and posttest period in fourteen of the fifteen categories of positive youth development we measured, while in most cases the comparison participants showed no change or declined in positive behavior and attitudes. We also accessed the court records of 200 clients and a random sample of 200 juveniles not in the PC&C program to measure recidivism, along with report cards of clients and comparison youth. Again the results were the same on the objective data. Recidivism rates declined significantly for the program clients and rose for the others. Report card grades rose significantly for the clients and remained much the same for the others.

While the evaluation was being conducted, another event related to PC&C found its way into the media. One of the ex-offenders had gotten involved in a serious situation where he appeared to be the victim. (Two years later it would be revealed that he was less a victim in this situation than was originally believed, but at the time of the press reports the PC&C employee was reported as the victim of the event.) This unfortunate event had the effect of reviving the battle of words between the directors of PC&C and the political leader. Media stories continued for weeks.

How did all the negative media coverage affect the evaluation and the daily work of the program? Actually, the effects were minimal. The program's director had been ordered by the executive director of the parent organization to refuse media interviews. We were too busy trying to follow this fast-moving program to consider the effects of the media coverage, as were most of the program staff. It was not until the week before I turned in the evaluation report that I began to feel pressure about the results. Just days before the report was due, I received a call from the new executive director of the parent agency, asking me to summarize the results. I did. He asked me if I had witnessed any questionable activity by the ex-offenders. I said that I had not. He then asked me if I would come before the organization's board and present the evaluation findings. I agreed to do this. He also added that he intended to do some reorganizing of the program.

The night I presented the findings to the board was one I must simply call surrealistic. Seated in the boardroom were board members representing various institutions and a few grassroots organizations, a staff member of the political leader that had opposed the program, the parent organization's new executive director, the newspaper reporter that had been covering the program controversies, and me. Board members had been given advance copies of the evaluation report. When I was introduced, a few board members commented that they had reviewed the report and thought it was very professional and reader friendly. I handed out tables and interactive graphs of every indicator category we measured, from each data source. One by one I showed them how the program clients had fared over the year, and how they compared to similar youths not in the program. Follow-up questions were few.

When my report was over, the organization's executive director passed out his reorganization plans. He began by stating that we had all probably been following the media reports and that he was in agreement with some of the criticism of the program and felt it was time to reorganize PC&C. He wished to eliminate the use of ex-offenders entirely, would be reassigning staff at all levels, would rename the program, and would eliminate all program activities that related to correctional facilities—field trips, collaborations, and sharing of resources. He presented flow charts and reorganization plans that moved the program away from its focus on crime prevention and more toward general youth development. I looked around the room for some board member ready to ask the obvious question: "Why are we trying to fix something that ain't broke?" but none materialized. I did observe expressions of confusion on the faces of some, but they did not speak up.

I left the meeting in a disorientated state. I had been in the field long enough to realize that evaluation reports (as well as needs assessments) rarely were used by organizational leaders to make major program changes or plan new activities (unless by some coincidence the reports recommended the changes the leaders were intending to make anyway). Lack of use of the evaluation did not surprise me. I knew (sadly) what was being suggested between the lines on this reorganization plan. The program's director would be fired or "reassigned," as would be some of the middle managers and all of the ex-offender staff. At that moment in the history of our firm, I believed this was the most favorable evaluation we had ever conducted. I did not feel overly surprised by the actions of the organization's new executive director. I believed there may have been things I did not know. Did he have some information I lacked? Had there been an incident with some staff that he and the board were keeping confidential? Might this have been an issue so serious that it suggested an entire reorganization of the program and its staff? Did the political leader that had opposed the program in the media convince the majority of the board that the program had to be reorganized, and was the executive director then simply under orders to do this? Might this have been an issue in his recent hiring? Or was he, as a new organizational leader, simply trying to end the negative media coverage? Did he design a reorganization plan to terminate the controversy over the hiring of the ex-offenders, hence ending the troublesome press coverage? I did not have the answers and do not to this day.

Before arriving at my office the next morning, the reporter covering the PC&C program had left a message asking me to call her. She said she was unclear about my evaluation findings and needed me to summarize them to her, as she wanted to get the story about the reorganization of PC&C in the next day's edition. I decided to take an hour to do some critical thinking. On the one hand, I visualized a headline reading something like: "PC&C Evaluation Outstanding, So Why Is Organization's Director Firing Staff, Reorganizing Program?" But I didn't believe this was about to happen. I had not seen any critical analysis of the PC&C controversy in her stories. She quoted the criticism of the political leader and the responses of the PC&C director, at least until the director was ordered to say nothing. PC&C staff said she had never visited the program. She had not created her own sources—she had simply repeated the information she was given. I did not expect any analysis of the situation.

Then that ugly question reared its head again. What, if anything, was my responsibility? Did I follow the old-school belief about evaluation and simply reiterate my findings, saying nothing at all to advocate for the program? Was my obligation to move far away from this detached point of view and advocate for the program, the way that some empowerment evaluation proponents suggest (Fetterman, 1994)? I came up with a plan. I would ask her what she thought.

I returned her call. The reporter asked me to summarize (in a concise and reader-friendly way) the results of the evaluation. I simply said, "I regard this program to be one of the top five programs we have ever evaluated in terms of positive outcomes, and it might just be number one." The reporter asked me how many programs I had evaluated. I said about forty (which was true at that time). She thanked me. I then initiated a conversation that went much like the following:

"What do you think this all means?"

"I'm not sure what you're getting at," responded the reporter.

"Why do you think they are reorganizing the program?"

"Well, probably because there's been some criticism," responded the reporter. The reporter then told me she had to get on with her story.

The following day the story appeared in the paper with a headline simply stating that the executive director of the large parent organization was reorganizing the PC&C program and would no longer hire ex-offenders or engage in work involving the correctional facilities. The reporter repeated the account of the past conflict between the program's directors and the political leader. In the second to last paragraph she mentioned that our firm had conducted a recent evaluation of the program. She did not include my remark about how positive the evaluation was relative to our other work, but instead added an anecdote I had mentioned in my presentation before the board. That was the end of the story.

Curiously, this program, like the immigrant gardens project, also had an interesting later development. In the weeks that followed the announcement of the program reorganization, the PC&C director was reassigned to a subordinate position and then quit. Nearly all the ex-offenders and some of the middle managers were also reassigned. Activities related in any way to correctional facilities were eliminated. The program was renamed. Several months passed and the program was up for annual re-funding. The proposal writers at the parent organization began the process of reapplying for funds from the governmental source that had been almost a sole supporter of PC&C during its long history. But the grant writers were confronted with quite a surprise when they began writing the reapplication and saw that the funding source only supported programs that were linked to correctional institutions, and hiring ex-offenders was a required component. The reorganization had removed the program from eligibility for the same funding that had kept it operating for all those years. The parent organization had to scamper to return some of the PC&C

components. A grant officer at the funding source, hearing news of the changes that had taken place, also issued a notice to the parent organization that the program needed to refocus its efforts on crime prevention again in order to be eligible for continuation of funds. Within a year some of the old staff returned, and the program looked much like it had when we first evaluated the effort.

Our firm was commissioned to do a follow-up study of PC&C three years later. The findings were nearly identical to the first evaluation. The political leader who had so criticized the effort had run into problems of his own and decided not to seek another elected term. With that, the media coverage of PC&C essentially ended (at least to the present date). How does it happen that the paper information lines can so miss the mark on social service programs?

THE STORY BEHIND THE STORIES

As was stated earlier, no objective news on these programs is simply out there to be gathered and published. All news has sources, and these sources are rarely media professionals gathering information on social programs on their own. Today, reporters rely more on news releases than ever before. Chris Frost (2002) in *Reporting for Journalists* described this growing tendency.

> The most common source of stories, certainly on local papers and local radio stations, is the press release. These have grown in importance over the last twenty years as editorial staffs in many provincial papers have been reduced and more and more organizations have become media sensitive. A local weekly paper that, during the 1970s, had an editorial staff of ten might now struggle by with five. . . . Whatever the reasons, newsdesks are now more likely to use press releases from local businesses, societies, sport clubs and am-dram groups than ever before. (p. 12)

Although instructional manuals and other publications are available to teach human service organizations how to use the media (e.g., Bonk, Griggs, & Tynes, 1999), in our experience, only the larger organizations actually have staff that can devote themselves to this activity. The more powerful sources are more likely to get their stories told. Large complex organizations, such as the lead agency in the REDUCE coalition, often have their own public relations people that know how to control the flow of information—either to see that the information does not get released or to control the kinds of information that do get released.

News releases in the form of public relations for program activities thus might find their way into the media through these sources. Headlines such as "Teens in Local Just Kids Program Learn Value of Volunteering" are not that uncommon. But what about more objective reports on these programs, say, from program evaluators? Evaluations of extremely large programs, such as national models with tens of thousands of participants (especially if these programs are controversial), might be published. But virtually never would a TV viewer or newspaper reader note a headline on an evaluation of a local, midsized program, and in those rare cases where this occurs, the press release often comes from the organizations being evaluated and only the positive findings are revealed. Program staff almost never send actual evaluation reports to the news media as press releases and the news media do not publish the results. Why is this? As confusing as this may sound, they do not do it because nobody does it. This brings us back to the theoretical foundations of hegemony and practice.

Recall the theory of hegemony from Chapter 1 (Gramsci, 1971). According to this theory, dominant groups in capitalist societies rule through special-purpose alliances. The alliances may include subordinate groups who negotiate their limited consent in return for getting some of their interests represented in the power bloc. Those interests might be resources allocated for social services. Hegemony also becomes a process of shaping ideology so the power of dominant groups appears natural and legitimate. Hegemony involves not only political and economic control, but also the ability of the dominant groups to project their own ways of representing the world, such as through the mass media. These representations are manifested as ideologies, or unconscious, taken-for-granted ideas embedded in material practices. The shaping of these ideologies entails both coercion and consent. The mass media play an important role in the shaping of this ideology, and some argue that at least a hint of coercion may be involved. Herbert Gans (1979) studied the way that network news and major news magazines decide what is news, and argued that journalists are "by no means free agents" (p. 235). News sources are more likely to be the most powerful public officials.

> Since the news media constitute their major communication
> outlet to the citizenry and are essential to the performance of
> their duties and the maintenance of their power, they would al-
> most certainly use that power to pressure the journalists were
> journalists to rely less upon them. (p. 282)

Political or other important leaders will usually have the ear of
members of the press. For example, it is unlikely that the PC&C program would ever have made front-page news had the program not
been singled out for criticism by the local political leader.

Others have argued that the media do not have an intentional bias
toward those in power, but end up demonstrating the bias in actual
practice. Goldman and Rajagopal (1991) posed an interesting question:

> How do the news media, while remaining independent from or-
> ganized political forces and engaged in no conspiracy to hood-
> wink the public, nonetheless regularly reproduce interpretations
> of events, which are consonant with the interests of dominant
> political and economic groups? (p. 20)

As was also mentioned in Chapter 1, the interests of subordinate
groups can at times be co-opted by more powerful partners in these
blocs. Recall the case of the immigrant gardens. The staff may have
wanted to garner media attention by organizing the gardeners against
the city government in protest of loss of the land, but they had to rely
on this same city government for their assets in other domains—their
office space and, more important, leases on vacant lots for other gardeners. The urban staff understood that they needed to preserve their
organization and program in order to serve the gardeners in any capacity. To preserve their organization, they needed to negotiate the
available land from the government.

Another argument often made by proponents of hegemony theory
is that the media, playing an integral role in the process of hegemony,
rarely report the news in terms of group or class interests. In discussing the media and the "ideological effect," Stuart Hall (1977, p. 336)
maintained that "the class nature of the state is masked: classes are re-
distributed into individual subjects: and these individuals are united
within the imaginary coherence of the state, the nation and the 'national interest.'" In most cases, consumers of social services are people of lower socioeconomic status, and monitoring of how their needs

are being met by social programs could be framed and represented as a class issue, but this is not done. Only rarely (e.g., when some organizational leader absconds with funds intended for the needy) do we find the media grasping at the story. The individual is highlighted. The lack of accountability mechanisms that allowed the leader to abscond with funds would not likely become the target of the story.

In all of these processes, the public comes to "understand" what is newsworthy and what is not. A public relations press release on a program event is newsworthy. An objective evaluation of the way the program is implemented and its outcomes is not. Recall also from Chapter 1 a discussion of Bourdieu's (1977) theory of practice. According to Bourdieu, patterns of practice, such as determining what is and is not newsworthy, emerge through historical and adaptive processes (such as those processes involved in the construction of hegemony). Over time the factors that led to these practices may be forgotten—a phenomenon he termed habitus. Individuals find themselves immersed in habitually and officially approved practices that begin to appear natural. Alternative courses of action appear unusual. A reader of the morning newspaper would not blink an eye over the headline and human interest story "Teens in Local Just Kids Program Learn Value of Volunteering," but the headline "Evaluation of Just Kids Program Had Mixed Results" is likely to generate some confusion. The reader might wonder: "Is there something about this program I should know—was it involved in some scandal?" "Does some celebrity run this program?" or "Is this some kind of program of massive size?" With this shared understanding through habitus, program and evaluation professionals rarely submit actual program evaluations (good or bad) as press releases, and when occasionally they do, journalists pretty much ignore them.

BUT THE STORY DOES NOT END HERE

Chapter 1 also emphasized the point that the theory of hegemony does not argue for any form of structural determinism. The theory points out ways that individuals and social groups can move beyond structural constraints and demystify ideology and reform systems. This is discussed in Chapter 7.

Before this discussion moves to the subject of change, as promised, I am going to shift gears and report on some of the best program efforts we have evaluated. The following chapter discusses factors that lead to well-implemented programs and often highly positive outcomes.

Chapter 5

The Other Side of the Page

It is time to turn the page. This book has dealt with accountability mechanisms in social services. The focus has been on accountability in program implementation, which involves two basic questions: (1) Does the program provide essentially the resources, services, and activities it has been funded to provide?* (2) What accountability mechanisms are in place to ensure this? I should note here that well-implemented programs do not necessarily translate into programs that achieve their anticipated outcomes. Any number of other factors can interfere with positive outcomes, such as faulty program models, turnover of key staff, or highly resistant clients. However, it has been our experience that well-implemented programs do usually produce at least some good outcomes for their consumers.

This chapter discusses well-implemented programs. In our fifty-plus program evaluations, most have been well implemented, and of these the overwhelming majority of programs have also had positive evaluation outcomes (those discussed here had excellent evaluation outcomes). Once again I repeat that if the reader experiences some surprise reading this book, it should not be that some programs are funded and yet never implemented per their stated objectives, but that so many programs are well implemented despite the dearth of accountability mechanisms.

In our experience, some factors lead to successful implementation. There is a small story here and a much bigger one.

---

*Program leaders often discover during early implementation stages that some changes need to be made, and it is not uncommon to notify funding agencies of the needed changes. Situations in which changes were made and the funding sources were notified of these changes can still be well-implemented programs.

doi:10.1300/5556_05

THE SMALL STORY:
THE NONDISCRETIONARY MODEL

Some programs have models that make it nearly impossible for staff to practice discretion in the services, activities, or resources they are supposed to provide. These are programs in which consumers can hold service providers accountable. In most cases, these programs and their resources are, first, well publicized (through Web sites, resource guides, referral sources, signage). The consumers and potential consumers know what these programs are supposed to offer. Second, these programs offer standardized services, activities, or resources. The consumers and potential consumers know what these programs are supposed to offer every time. Third, these programs have stable program sites. The consumers and potential consumers know exactly where to go to access these services, activities, or resources—or to make complaints about lack of access. Fourth, these programs have places where consumers can gather en masse (as opposed to being served individually). The consumers and potential consumers can check with each other to see if resources are being uniformly distributed; they can make public complaints causing at minimum some embarrassment to neglectful staff; and they can organize in groups to make complaints to those ostensibly responsible for ensuring appropriate service (e.g., supervisors, parent organizations, funding sources).

Many community centers fit into this paradigm. For example, it would be hard to imagine staff at a community center making a discretionary decision not to open a swimming pool at the hours advertised on brochures and Web sites when they knew that scores of consumers would be at the door demanding the promised pool services.

The urban gardens program discussed in Chapter 4 is another example of the nondiscretionary model. Consumers rented garden plots at stable sites in the presence of other consumers. Signage and brochures informed them of the services and supplies they would receive with their plots. At their plots, the consumers also gardened next to other consumers. If a neglectful staff member had failed to provide one gardener with some supply, the consumer would quickly note that the other gardeners had it and could return to the rental office to issue a complaint in the presence of others about the discrepancy.

The nondiscretionary program model works because consumers clearly know what resources, services, and activities are supposed to be provided under all circumstances. However, most human services cannot operate under the "one size fits all" paradigm. Human needs and social problems are complex and require programming that is tailored to meet the more specific needs of individuals and groups. That brings us to the bigger picture.

THE BIG STORY: ETHICS-BASED LEADERSHIP

Susan Schissler Manning (2003) has written an outstanding and comprehensive volume on ethical leadership in human services. In this work she discussed multiple dimensions of ethical leadership, including the dual private and public responsibilities of human service workers. According to the author, the private duty that human service professionals have involves a client-first orientation and competency. Commitment to clients and competence are central to the National Association of Social Workers' code of ethics (1996; see also Reamer, 1998).

> Professionals must be trustworthy in order to have moral authority. The trustworthiness of a professional is based on having the best interests of clients at heart, which translates into real action, not just rhetoric, on behalf of clients. . . . The ethical mandate then, for social workers and other professions with private duties (for example, medicine, psychology, or nursing) is to be competent in their occupational duty, serve according to a professional code of ethics, and ensure that service delivered and agency practices are in the best interests of the consumers of service. (Manning, 2003, p. 11)

The public duty of human service professionals is described as "making the invisible visible."

> [Human service] professionals act as the *public custodian*, nurturing and interpreting the basic values of society. Values, such as social justice, access to health care, civil liberties, fairness in the distribution of benefits and burdens, economic considerations, and so forth are examples of the moral issues that are promulgated or shaped through professional human services.

... This duty to the public interest provides accurate information to policymakers, citizens, and other interested parties about the state of our social welfare and human service system. In the process, values of social justice, self-determinism, and altruism are asserted into the public dialogue. This duty can only be enhanced through effective leadership and ethical organizational structures. A leader's ability to create and maintain communication with direct service workers; consumers of services; and social, political, and economic representatives in the community becomes the highway for "making the invisible visible" to society. (Manning, 2003, pp. 11-12)

Manning also discussed three attributes and characteristics of ethical leadership in human service. The first is "sacrifice," which "provides the most clear and evident moral voice to constituents" (p. 64). This includes sacrifice of one's own time and resources and can even include willingness to sacrifice employment if one is coerced into participation in an unethical practice. Manning's second characteristic is a "voice of conscience" within organizations, which involves continually advocating for ethical practices and having the courage to publicly resist unethical practices. The third characteristic is "craft and competence." This characteristic includes one's own competence but also attention to the competence of others.

The leader consciously communicates an unwillingness to accept inept or incompetent performance from constituents in the organization. The work with constituents through the relationships and interactions of the organizational community influences leaders and constituents to develop a consciousness of craft in the organization. (Manning, 2003, p. 67)

In nearly all of the well-implemented projects that have been evaluated by Jill Florence Lackey & Associates, we have encountered program leaders with most of the attributes and sense of duty described. Following are a few examples.

PC&C: How the Stepford Staff Came to Be

Recall the case of the Preventing Crime and Corrections (PC&C) program. This program was well implemented and produced outstanding evaluation outcomes. The evaluation team from Jill Florence Lackey & Associates coined the phrase "the Stepford staff" because the program's personnel (particularly the middle managers) seemed almost too perfect to be real. In that program I was observing Rogell, a middle manager whose main responsibility was working with and supervising staff that referred youths from the courtrooms into community service and other PC&C activities. The PC&C program was located in a building several miles away from the parent organization's central offices, and staff had minimal interaction with staff from the central office or other programs (although they were housed in a building with other programs). They spent their days (and often their nights) with their clients, the families of the clients, and other PC&C staff. In the process of evaluating the program, I learned that Rogell was the only staff member who had been with the program since its inception over fifteen years earlier. Rogell would open the PC&C office each morning at 7:00 (although he did not get paid for any extra hours he worked), and during the season when the program's basketball leagues were competing, he would work many nights until midnight. He had quietly set a standard for other staff and over the years a program subculture of high achievement and client-centeredness had developed.

Rogell had worked under a series of directors—some who were involved in the media battles described in the previous chapter. Rogell himself had never served as the director, although for a brief time he was promoted to a "codirector" position. I never learned why he did not serve in the top program position, but I had a few clues from interview findings. One day I was attempting to tape record an interview with Rogell in his office. We were continually interrupted by phone calls from clients, client families, and collaborators—an angry mother wanting to know why her son had to write a letter to the judge, a client saying he could not find the address of his community service referral, the community service referral wondering what had happened to the youth offender. Between phone calls, I asked him, "Why have you done this all these years?"

Rogell smiled in his melancholy way and replied, "Jill, I took this job more than fifteen years ago. From the very first day I knew this was all I was ever going to want to do." He told me that I would see what an impact the program had on the kids when all my "statistics were in."

This mother here, she called me and she chewed me out because she thinks we shouldn't have her kid writing a letter to the judge explaining what he did wrong. She'll see. Years and years later these kids, and their parents, come back. Some of them work for the program now. They will remember all they had to go through here to make amends to the victims and all—to take responsibility for their actions. But they go out and become good citizens. Two-thirds do every year and we know this.

When I interviewed the six staff that worked under Rogell, opinions on his leadership style were mixed. Three praised him. "He's all for our kids," remarked one staff member. "And he's for the community. He doesn't want one of our kids going out and making some member of our community a victim again."

The other three found Rogell overly taxing and complained strongly to members of the evaluation team about him. The remarks of one young woman typified the comments of those who considered him demanding:

I don't think he has any leadership skills at all. He thinks that we should come to these championship games when our kids play in them. That's too much. He might be a twenty-four/seven kind of guy, but I put in a hard day and my own time is my own time. I'm happy for our kids, but my job stops at five. Where's the concern for us? He doesn't know how to lead his staff, and he isn't a good boss.

When I returned to evaluate this program again three years later, the three staff that found fault with Rogell's "demands" had left and the other three were still with the program. A member of the latter group had been promoted to a middle manager. Over the years, Rogell's client- and community-centered approach had taken hold through a process of "natural selection." New program directors came and went, but the line staff had their own subculture.

PC&C was a program of substantial size, with twenty-one staff. Read on for another well-implemented program with only two staff.

No-Place-Like-Home: Men on a Mission

Two formerly homeless men operated the "No-Place-Like-Home" program, which provided resources to the currently homeless through a well-stocked mobile van. The two men had actually founded the program. When they were successful in getting off the streets, they approached a large nonprofit organization sponsoring programs for the homeless, claiming that many of the homeless did not use shelters and as such had no access to the resources and referrals that would help them solve their problems and find permanent housing. The nonprofit saw an opportunity to implement the program by finding a legislator that would propose legislation to support it. Located in the legislator's district was a day center for the homeless with potential voters. The legislator collaborated with the advocates for the homeless, the nonprofit, the homeless themselves, and other legislators. This newly created alliance was able to achieve its aims and the program was funded and later implemented.

The goals of the implemented program were to assist people who were currently homeless and to provide counseling and referrals that would help them get off the streets. Items the homeless could access from the van included blankets, food, clothing, toiletries, lists of helping agencies and resources, books, paper and pencils, shoes, calendars, lists of available job openings, and pamphlets on health issues and safety. The van was also equipped with hotlines so that the staff could call shelters, clinics, and other agencies to arrange for appointments and referrals for the homeless. The program appeared so popular with the homeless that other nonprofits began to duplicate it. Soon three mobile programs were operating out of vans in the same urban area.

Our firm was commissioned to conduct a low-budget evaluation of this project because grant officers from their governmental funding source had expressed concerns that there were too many mobile homeless services (all operating out of vans) in this city and the officers were considering dropping some of them. Thus one of our evaluation roles was to discover if there was something unique about this program that made it less of a duplication of services.

There was. The homeless actually used this service.

We knew the No-Place-Like-Home project was unique before we actually began the evaluation. In every case where it is possible, our firm preresearches programs before finalizing any evaluation models or before we begin developing measurement instruments. During our preresearch visit to one of the sites where the van was parked, we noticed the obvious. The line for services at the No-Place-Like-Home van was twelve deep, despite the fact that two blocks away (and in easy sight of these homeless people) was another mobile service unit with no line. I went to visit the other van and discovered that most of the same resources were offered these. My interest immediately transcended simply evaluating outcomes and turned to understanding why the homeless were making considerably more use of the No-Place-Like-Home service.

During the following week I rode in the van with the staff. For the first two days, the staff may have been somewhat intimidated by my presence and rarely said anything to me. Everywhere they stopped, they knew the homeless people by name. They handed out whatever material needs were requested, but also continued an ongoing yet very discreet and sensitive dialogue with each homeless person. They asked how an injury was healing, if someone had gotten treatment for an infection, how the temporary job worked out, how someone was handling an issue involving substance use, if someone had taken advantage of free HIV testing, whether a shelter referral was needed, and on and on. Even in my presence, the homeless people spoke to them frankly about their current status and experiences. Some of the conversations focused on substance use, and they tended to unfold something like the following:

STAFF MEMBER: Did you need a shelter referral, "James"?

HOMELESS MAN: No, the blanket's fine. The weather's good. I didn't go to that meeting like you suggested, but I read the stuff you gave me.

STAFF MEMBER: When you want to talk, we're here.

HOMELESS MAN: Bro—I know that. You guys been good to me. I know what I gotta do. I just gotta wait for my time.

STAFF MEMBER: You need to have faith that your time will come. We know it will.

After the first two days, the No-Place-Like-Home staff began to talk to me about their program. These two gentlemen had always been the program's only staff. They were homeless themselves for over ten years before they went into recovery for crack cocaine addictions. They discussed the number of homeless people that remained on the streets because of addictions. "Sometimes they started using something after they got homeless because they lost hope," one said.

"We just try and talk to them—let them know that they can just be honest with us and we are there for them, to guide them into treatment, if they ever choose it." The main issue they continued to stress was how street life increased substance use and abuse, and how programs needed to make efforts to keep people from becoming homeless in the first place, rather than just supplying emergency services to those who were already homeless.

Then at the end of the week, the two staff requested a favor. Very hesitantly, they asked me if I might develop a survey for them to administer to find out how much substance abuse had changed for their clients after they became homeless. I said I certainly would do this as a personal favor. They also asked me to keep it private—not to tell the parent organization that they were going to conduct this survey. I asked why and they simply said that they had brought the idea to their agency's administrators in the past and the idea had been rejected as irrelevant to their program, as their program was not focused on homelessness prevention. I developed the survey immediately for the staff.

In the next several months we completed the evaluation. Our evaluation team conducted qualitative interviews, observation, and a retrospective pre- and posttest survey with homeless and formerly homeless clients who used the No-Place-Like-Home mobile services exclusively and other homeless clients who used alternative mobile services (as a comparison group). In terms of getting off the streets, finding employment, reducing substance use, maintaining healthy habits, and forging ties in the community, the outcomes were significantly more favorable for those using the No-Place-Like-Home services than the comparison group. Findings from the qualitative data strongly suggested that the staff's personal contact with the homeless, development of trusting relationships, and keeping an eye on their daily needs and activities played key roles in the more successful outcomes for this mobile service. When the parent organization received the report, administrators requested that this finding be deleted, citing "boundary issues." They said that they expected the staff to maintain a professional distance from their clientele. As a compromise I deleted a few words, but I left that finding essentially in place. The favorable evaluation of this project, however, did nothing to maintain its funding. With evaluation in hand, but likely never read, the governmental funding source cut all funds for the program. Fortunately, within weeks a grant from a private funding source came through and the program remained intact.

What happened to the survey the program's staff had requested? Eighteen months after completing this evaluation, our firm was evaluating another homeless-serving program in the same city. I attended a small meeting with representatives of homeless-serving organizations and a local funding agency. At the meeting, several organizational directors were discussing an "anonymous survey" that had been conducted and the results mailed to them. According to the anonymous researchers, over 70 percent of people on the streets reported increased substance use after becoming homeless. The one-page report listed some of the actual survey questions—thus I knew it was the survey I developed for the No-Place-Like-Home staff. The actual reason that these directors mentioned the survey was to figure out who would have conducted the survey and why the source needed to be anonymous. However, once that topic was explored, several people at the table did mention that their own staff had discussed this substance-using tendency before. Hence, they asked each other if there might be something to the finding. The leader of the funding agency said that homelessness prevention might be something that needed more attention in this city. This discussion continued into several other meetings.

During the year that we conducted the evaluation of this second homeless-serving agency, I noticed the topic of substance abuse among the homeless coming up almost routinely. Whether the new-found interest in the topic was generated by that survey is not known. Nor was it known if the interest would eventually find its way into new homelessness prevention programming in the city. But it is surely possible that a relatively invisible local problem had been made more visible by the work of two highly motivated street workers.

In the past two examples, individuals with the leadership attributes and the dual sense of duty discussed by Manning (2003) led the programs. Read on for a case in which the organizational leadership set the tone for an exemplary program.

The A-JOB Program: "Let's Get Real"

Our firm was contacted to evaluate a program for a small organization called "Economic Initiative, Inc." Economic Initiative ran three programs with twelve staff. One program organized businesses in the central city to expand resources and effect policies that would keep these resources in the area; another was a job training program ("A-JOB"); and the third was a counseling program designed to help central city residents become economically self-sufficient.

A man and a woman codirected Economic Initiative. The pair had left work in the private and public sector after growing frustrated with the lack of positive outcomes in programs they had worked for. The woman codirector, whom I will call "Alicia," was a psychotherapist who had been employed in a private, for-profit counseling firm. In our first meeting, she told me that the firm she left seemed more oriented toward retaining clients (and the insurance money they brought in) than actually helping these clients. "There was too much enabling people with bad habits," she argued. Alicia said that often the psychotherapist knew after a few meetings that a client's feelings of exhaustion or lack of self-worth were probably due more to a lack of initiative—failure to set and meet goals—than to external factors. When she tried to work with these clients to take more initiative and stop blaming others, the clients would sometimes request another therapist and Alicia would be called in to her supervisor to explain what went wrong. "The message I was consistently given, albeit subtly, was to find a way to assure the clients that their problems were never their own fault." Alicia looked for a way to strike out on her own.

Some years later she met "Rodney" at a community meeting. Rodney was complaining at the meeting about the lack of positive outcomes that needy men were having in a central city job-training program, for which he worked. "This program was basically teaching people skills that the staff had—not what would get the clients jobs." He said that the program leaders basically hired their friends, and one friend was an unemployed graphic artist. The graphic artist taught the clients how to design ads, knowing what he already knew—that any opening for a graphic artist in the city would be met by hundreds of résumés, and most of the applicants would have actual experience and degrees in the field. Rodney said he felt a moral obligation to offer training in occupations that were actually needed.

After meeting for about a year, Alicia and Rodney teamed up to develop Economic Initiative, Inc. They said they had a "let's get real" attitude from the start. They began by conducting a needs assessment of businesses in the central city. They learned that two trades in greatest demand were welding and printing. Hence they developed a program to train central city residents in these skills.

Alicia and Rodney also wished to stress duties over rights across their three programs. They emphasized this through a series of pacts. In the business collaboration program, the staff and directors from Economic Initiative signed pacts indicating it was their duty to work to expand resources and effect public policy that would keep businesses economically viable in the city, but that the business owners in exchange had to sign pacts outlining their duties to their employees (e.g., family-supporting wages, health insurance, good working conditions, equitable employment practices). In the job-training program, the staff signed a pact indicating they would train clients in skills that would actually result in job offers, and they would work with the industries to ensure fair labor policies. The clients in turn signed pacts that they had duties to the employers, which included steady attendance, positive attitudes, and productive work habits. Staff in the counseling program signed a pact that they would help the clients to become economically self-sufficient through strategies proven to work through rigorous evaluation. Counseling clients then had the duty to follow through with the practices—for the sake of their families, friends, and the larger community.

The codirectors admitted that they had difficulty getting their programs to run efficiently during the first few years. "We expected our staff to honor the same sense of duty that they were teaching their clients," said Rodney. "If a welding teacher shows up late for class, he will not last here. How can we teach potential workers to be on time at the job if our trainers are not on time?" Over the years, the organization went through the same process of natural selection as some of the programs described earlier did, and by the end of the decade they had developed a subculture of high achievement and a strong sense of duty within the small organization.

Our firm evaluated the A-JOB (Accessing Jobs by Overcoming Barriers) program. The program had three components. The first was a "soft skills" training program. Here counselors from the organization's economic counseling program took A-JOB clients on a week-long retreat where the clients were counseled in taking responsibility for their own actions in their families and communities, and in their duties toward fair employers. The second component was an eight-week skills training program in welding or printing. The final component was an eight-week internship in a local industry in one of these two occupational areas. During this time, the employer could also assess the quality of the intern's work to determine whether this individual was appropriate for the company. The program, after a decade of refinement, was nearly flawlessly implemented. We followed the progress of their clients vis-à-vis potential clients on a waiting list (the comparison group). In all areas measured over a two-year period—job retention, income, benefits, sense of personal satisfaction, family relations, economic self-sufficiency, community relations—the clients showed significant improvements over time and significantly more improvements than members of the comparison group.

The programs outlined in this section were stellar efforts. But before the reader becomes too optimistic in believing one can know just how to ensure a successful program, some limitations need to be discussed.

A WORD ABOUT GOOD LEADERSHIP

First of all, the reader might wonder why the examples focused on both program leaders and organizational leaders. Might it make more sense if organizations put maximum effort into hiring organizational directors with all the leadership qualities outlined by Manning (2003) and then allowed the process of natural selection to ensue? Might a subculture of deeply committed action be more likely to emerge from the top than the bottom?

Although rigorous research needs to be done on the subject, from my perspective, the issue seems to be limited by scope. The larger the organization, the more difficult it becomes for an ethical leader or leaders to maintain a subculture that is both client centered and public centered. For example, over the years Jill Florence Lackey & Associates has evaluated three programs for one very large social service agency. The executive director of this agency has consistently held a reputation of being a visionary leader with a strong sense of altruism. However, as the agency grew, the attention of the director and the administrative staff necessarily turned to maintaining the agency and the programs under its umbrella. The administrative staff under the executive director were necessarily preoccupied with bureaucratic maintenance, proposal writing (and other forms of fund-raising), employee relations, and collaborators within the human service industry. The altruistic tendencies of the director moved from concern about the clients, whom he no longer saw, to concern about maintaining his staff and collaborators, whom he often saw at regular intervals. In the three programs we evaluated for this agency, only one was well implemented (yet lacked favorable outcomes due to a program model that failed to match the needs of the clientele). Another of this agency's efforts was a paper program in that the staff rarely even came to work, much less serving the clients its formal records claimed. Another had implemented about half of its officially stated activities, services, and resources and had some positive program outcomes. Wheatley and Kellmer-Rogers (1999) described the process of losing the initial vision:

> We see the depths of passion whenever an organization invites its people to create a vision. . . . We create an organization. People who loved the purpose of an organization grow to disdain the institution that was created to fulfill it. Passion mutates into procedures, into rules and roles. Instead of purpose we focus on policies. Instead of being free to create, we impose constraints that squeeze the life out of us. (p. 57)

In our experience, the subculture of service involving self-sacrifice, client centeredness, a sense of public duty, and an insistence on competence begins to dissipate when employee numbers grow. The PC&C program, with twenty-one staff, was the largest program we ever evaluated where this subculture clearly was manifested.

But does stellar programming not in some way reflect policies of the parent organization and, most particularly, the leaders of the parent organization? Is there something about PC&C and the commitment of its twenty-one "Stepford staff" that reflected positive enabling policies of the organization's leaders? Or, to put this another way, was there something about a paper program like PAY, where most clients existed in falsified case management records only, that reflected negative enabling policies of the organization's leaders? Well, actually not. You see, PC&C and PAY were both programs of the City Life Institute. The two programs ran concurrently, out of the same building, and under the umbrella of the same parent agency. Many of the answers still appear to lie with the accountability mechanisms.

THE STORY DOES NOT END HERE

This chapter has discussed two factors that can lead to successful implementation of programs. One is the nondiscretionary model in which programs are well publicized (through Web sites, resource guides, referral sources, signage); offer standardized services, activities, or resources; have stable program sites; and have places where consumers can gather in groups rather than being served individually. But this chapter also acknowledged that a "one size fits all" program does not often address issues involved in complex human and social problems.

This chapter then described the other factor that can lead to successful program implementation—ethics-based leadership. I cannot overemphasize the importance of this factor. This leadership model involves a private sense of duty toward clients, a public sense of duty toward the general community, and attributes of sacrifice, a voice of conscience, and competence at all service levels. Although this leadership model is clearly demonstrated in the best of our own program evaluations, it is one that is sometimes difficult to maintain.

First, in each of the case studies, the leaders had longevity in the programs. They went through years of retaining staff with similar commitments while easing out those that did not share these attributes. But unfortunately, few human service staff are able to remain in programs that long. One of the main reasons for staff turnover is the fluctuation in funding sources. Most nongovernmental social service programs run on "soft money" and must survive from grant to grant. A cut in funds for any reason can eliminate key positions in one sweeping move, irrespective of the quality of the personnel.

Second—and to be frank—not all social service professionals are willing (or able) to make the kind of sacrifices needed to fulfill the model of ethics-based leadership. They are confronted with competing demands, perhaps from family members, friends, or even other worthy causes that they may be championing in their free time. They may not have the financial security to make decisions such as surrendering their positions if unethical practices arise in their organizations.

Finally, we have found a number of cases in which administrators of social service agencies actually discourage staff who are willing to sacrifice on behalf of the clients or the public. We have evaluated programs whose personnel complain that they are discouraged from putting in unpaid overtime to help clients. In some cases, the administrative leaders may be suspicious of the motives of the staff and fear legal consequences. But in most cases, administrative leaders claim that they worry that program success will be too contingent on the presence of particular staff, or they fear that this kind of leadership will set consumer expectations too high if these staff are lost.

Although ethics-based leadership is so much a part of the equation, the need still exists to increase accountability mechanisms. Before exploring ways that this might be done, the reader needs to know more about the process of evaluating programs in the real world. Before evaluators should be considered as mainstays in increasing accountability in the human service industry, the reader should understand the needs for reform in this practice.

Chapter 6

The Role Evaluators Can Play,
and Why We So Seldom Do

The practice of program evaluation emerged during the late 1960s. This field of scientific inquiry followed the development of many Great Society programs of the Johnson administration and the concern expressed by some governmental and private agencies that there be a way of holding the new programs accountable for the use of public money and delivery of promised services. Since that time, the field has grown significantly. Although there is no way of knowing how many evaluators practice today, Rossi, Freeman, and Lipsey (1999) estimated that the number in the United States alone might be as high as 50,000 or even double or triple that. Of these practitioners, Rossi et al. pointed out that only a few thousand belong to professional membership organizations such as the American Evaluation Association or attend annual conferences of these organizations. A quick glance at the published works on evaluation will reveal that at least eight in ten authors list their primary associations as colleges or universities. Most of these faculty also teach, as opposed to working at university research centers. Few of the academically based evaluators rely on grant money from program evaluation for their day-to-day livelihood, and when they do, the grant money is usually secured independently of the programs being evaluated. Many of these academically based evaluators also design their own programs and then secure grant money to operate and self-evaluate the programs.

This arrangement is not the norm in the field. I wish to distinguish the academically based practitioners from what I term "ground-level" program evaluators. Ground-level evaluators comprise the overwhelming majority of the estimated 50,000 to 150,000 practitioners. They are evaluators who may be (1) associated with nonprofit or for-profit

doi:10.1300/5556_06

research firms, (2) working as private consultants in evaluation, or (3) employed to conduct evaluations by the parent organizations of the programs being evaluated (or at minimum, have the evaluation role listed among other roles in their job descriptions). As Weiss (1987) stated, "evaluation is generally commissioned by the agency responsible for the program, not the recipients of its efforts" (p. 59). This group of evaluators might work at evaluation part time or full time, have varying skills and training in evaluation research, and may move fluidly in and out of the field—but nearly all will share one common constraint: All are highly dependent on the program being evaluated for their means of production. Most of the time they rely on the program (or the program's parent organization) for their evaluation agreements (whether these are contracts with outside evaluators or job descriptions for internal evaluators), payments, approval of designs and methods, access to clients and other program stakeholders, and access to program records. As evaluation was first emerging as a practice in its own right, published literature did tend to raise questions about the relationship of evaluation sponsors and evaluators. In the following quote, Scriven (1983) discusses a "managerial ideology" as it relates to the role of both external and internal program evaluators:

> When program evaluation began to emerge, who commissioned it? Program instigators and managers, legislators and program directors. And whose programs were being evaluated? Programs initiated by the same legislators and managers. It is hardly surprising that a bias emerged from this situation. In the boldest economic terms, the situation could often be represented in the following way: someone looking for work as an evaluator (e.g., bidding on an evaluation contract) knew that they could not in the long run survive from the income from one contract. It followed that it was in their long-term self-interest to be doing work that would be attractive to the agency letting the contract. Since that agency was typically also the agency responsible for the program, it also followed [that] the evaluators understood that favorable reports were more likely to be viewed as good news than unfavorable ones.
>
>   . . . When we move further down the spectrum [speaking of internal evaluators], to the usual situation in a school district where the Title I evaluator may be on the staff of the Title I

projects manager, the pressures toward a favorable report become extreme. Everyone knows of cases where the project manager simply removes the critical paragraphs from the evaluator's report and sends it on upstairs as a co-authored evaluation. (pp. 232-233)

Today, little has changed in the field, but very few publications on evaluation mention the conflict of interest apparent when evaluation sponsors (those paying the bills) are over and over again the organizations and programs being evaluated. In an edited volume titled *Responding to Sponsors and Stakeholders in Complex Evaluation Environments,* the volume's editors sum up the chapter authors' perspectives on stakeholder issues with the following carefully written statement (Bernstein, Whitsett, & Mohan, 2002):

Some may question the importance, or even the reality of "objectivity." Be that as it may, many evaluators, particularly those trained as auditors, and many evaluation clients may feel that an evaluator's work is strengthened when the evaluation maintains an objective perspective, is seen by others as independent and objective, and when the evaluator's interaction with sponsors and stakeholders does not compromise his or her independence. (pp. 95-96)

The seemingly guarded choice of words here may simply reflect the fact that few researchers that publish often on program evaluation face the daily constraints of sponsorship (because most of those who publish are academics whose primary role is teaching, and they only occasionally hold contracts from the same organizations they are to evaluate). Or the careful wording may be due to growing trends in evaluation practice that tend to give increasing power to the evaluation clients/sponsors (e.g., Patton, 1997; Fetterman, 1996), as discussed in Chapter 2.

Whatever the reason for the lack of attention to possible conflicts of interest in the published evaluation literature, sponsorship constraints are issues that ground-level evaluators face daily. This concern for "clientism" is reflected in section E4 of the Guiding Principles for Evaluators of the American Evaluation Association (1995), and the wording could surely be strengthened.

Evaluators should maintain a balance between client needs and other needs. Evaluators necessarily have a special relationship with the client who funds or requests the evaluation. By virtue of that relationship, evaluators must strive to meet legitimate client needs whenever it is feasible and appropriate to do so. However, that relationship can also place evaluators in difficult dilemmas when client interests conflict with other interests, or when client interests conflict with the obligation of evaluators for systematic inquiry, competence, integrity, and respect for people. (p. 25)

The ultimate dependence on the program being evaluated holds the potential to color every process described in this chapter. But before I discuss these ubiquitous influences in the "real practicing world," I would like to describe an ideal evaluation process. The process described next actually unfolds on occasion for ground-level evaluators, albeit rarely.

THE IDEAL CIRCUMSTANCES
FOR EFFECTIVE EVALUATION PRACTICE

Ideal circumstances for evaluation must begin during the program planning process. This planning process precedes program implementation and often precedes program funding.

Pre-Program Planning

In an ideal situation, the evaluator is brought into the process as a new program is being planned. In this scenario, program developers have reliable needs assessment data identifying community needs and the developers design the program to meet those needs. At this time, the evaluator works with the program developers and all other relevant stakeholders, such as program collaborators and consumers/clients, to help clarify what the program expects to accomplish (House, 2003; Owen & Rogers, 1999; Rutman, 1980). The first question to be answered is: Does this program carry the potential to meet the needs identified by the needs assessment? If not, the effort requires redesigning. If yes, evaluators can help developers with program clarification processes through a variety of formats including diagrams or narrative descriptions that chart out the assumptions and processes inherent in the program design. The diagrams, sometimes referred to as *logic models,* might simply be flow charts, provide "if-then" sequences, or focus on inputs, outputs, and outcomes (changes in actual behavior or structures) and impacts (far-reaching changes in lifestyle and the community at large). Figure 6.1 is a hypothetical example of how the No-Place-Like-Home program might have looked in this format.

In collaboration with the program developers and other stakeholders, the evaluator then can develop an evaluation plan to measure progress on the inputs, outputs, and outcomes. Measurements of progress on inputs and outputs are often called *process evaluations* or *formative evaluations.* This kind of evaluation focuses on the implementation of the program and the ways that it operates on a daily basis. Measurements of progress on outcomes and impacts are often called (appropriately) *outcome* or *impact evaluations* or *summative evaluations.* When Jill Florence Lackey & Associates holds a multiyear contract to evaluate a specific program, it is not uncommon for us to conduct these two types of evaluations separately.

In an ideal situation, the evaluator will spend considerable time with program stakeholders (always including potential program consumers), giving them information about various evaluation types, genres, models, and methods, and explaining what each accomplishes and the strengths and weaknesses of each. This way the stakeholders can be active and informed participants in helping to create the

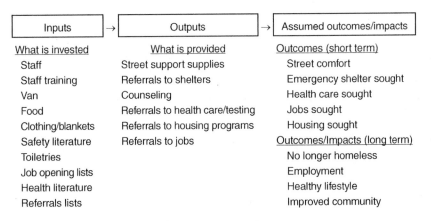

FIGURE 6.1. Hypothetical example of No-Place-Like-Home program.

evaluation plan. Under both ideal and nonideal circumstances, the evaluation plan should end up including mixed methods to strengthen the overall design, with the selection of methods driven by the evaluation questions being asked (Creswell, 2003). As Rossi et al. (1999) state, "the use of multiple methods, often referred to as *triangulation,* can strengthen the validity of findings if results produced by different methods are congruent" (p. 423).

In ideal circumstances, experimental or quasi-experimental designs are presented to the stakeholders as the best options for measurements of outcomes or impacts (see more on this in Chapter 2). The evaluator might make this recommendation for the same reasons given by Crane (1998) in his work in setting assessment criteria for determining effective social programs:

> A pure experimental design in which evaluation participants are randomly assigned to treatment and control groups is the universally accepted gold standard in evaluation research. Results generated from studies using this design have a lot of credibility, although even they may suffer from problems such as attrition bias or issues of external validity. When random assignment is not feasible, evaluators typically select a comparison group, using any one of a number of techniques designed to make it as similar as possible to the treatment population [a quasi-experimental design]. (p. 4)

From time to time and for various reasons, involved program stakeholders might tell the evaluator that they do not want an experimental or quasi-experimental design. The evaluator may then alter the design and try to add additional data sources and methods to strengthen the study.

The next process in the ideal scenario during the pre-program planning stage is to exchange some form of memorandum of understanding (MOU)—an agreement from the evaluator that he or she will conduct the evaluation if and when the program begins, and an agreement from program developers that this evaluator will be used to evaluate the program. The program developers then write proposals to seek funding sources for the program, if funding is not already available. The evaluator may then write the evaluation section of the proposal.

Program Implementation Stage

In an ideal situation, the evaluator is notified the very minute a program begins implementation. At this point, formal agreements are usually made and all details finalized (e.g., contracts with external evaluators). The early start enables the evaluator to randomly assign program participants to the intervention (treatment) and control groups, if a pure experimental design is used, or begin constructing a comparison group, if a quasi-experimental design is used.

The evaluator will collect process data during the implementation period to determine whether program inputs (such as staff and training) are in place and whether these inputs are resulting in the program services, activities, and resources expected (the outputs). A competent evaluator will use any combination of qualitative and quantitative data (such as observation or client satisfaction surveys) to measure these processes. In an ideal setting, feedback from evaluation data occurs at regular intervals and frequently. The evaluator works diligently to maintain relaxed and amicable relationships with all program stakeholders. In my experience, effective feedback should always begin with and focus on the positives. Wherever negative findings must be discussed, these findings should be steeped in data from multiple sources, and even then the results should be described in the most diplomatic terms possible. I have known evaluation practitioners I would describe as "gotcha" people, and they rarely encourage program leaders to modify program shortcomings.

The early stages often yield information that suggests some needed changes. For example, our firm conducted a process evaluation of a newly implemented program where computer instructors would teach central city high school students how to use some of the most sophisticated (and newly developed) software. The program was planned in response to a local business survey indicating that the young people most likely to be hired out of high school were those that knew the latest software programs. The program was designed to have trainers from the software programs first coach the computer instructors, and then the instructors were to teach the students.

However, as the program unfolded, the computer instructors were teaching the students the more traditional software programs and only introducing them to the capacity of the newer programs. The instructors did not see this as a problem because they did not realize that the program had been developed to help get students jobs with the skills specifically mentioned by the business respondents. Evaluation observation and interviews confirmed that the trainers from the software programs had provided faulty and incomplete information to the instructors on the software programs, and once the computer instructors were left on their own, many times they could not even open the new programs.

A major input had not been properly implemented (training); thus a major output did not materialize (instructors teaching students the latest software). Because the program supervisors were not on-site to observe either the initial training or the program, they did not actually know that the youths were not learning the latest software. Feedback from the process evaluation then resulted in retraining of the computer instructors.

Program Outcome Stage

In an ideal situation, all implementation problems have been addressed early in the program's history, and the outcome/impact evaluation will end up measuring what it is supposed to measure—whether or not the program model is actually accomplishing what it was set up to accomplish. In my experience, most well-implemented programs do accomplish at least some of their anticipated outcomes or impacts. There is almost always something in the findings that requires some level of change or improvement—whether it is program intensity, unclear roles or unevenness in performance of staff, high attrition rates, inadequate facilities, unclear documentation—and these issues again should be communicated in the most diplomatic ways possible, with the emphasis on the positives. In the ideal situation, the written and oral outcome report is reviewed by all involved stakeholders, and the evaluator is able to remain with the program long enough to attend (or even host) meetings to plan changes, if needed, in response to the evaluation findings. Finally, in the ideal situation, the suggested changes are actually made.

In this scenario, evaluation plays a very strong role in helping programs reach their maximum effectiveness and providing an assurance that a paper program will not result. However, the number of times that I personally have evaluated programs where these circumstances existed can be counted on one hand. The circumstances fail to materialize for complex reasons, which cannot be blamed on one situation, one process, or one person. The failures occur all the way through the system.

WHY BEST PRACTICES IN EVALUATION RARELY OCCUR

The demands for evaluation have increased in recent decades. The 1993 Government Performance and Results Act (GPRA) as well as the initiative of United Way of America have urged programs to focus on evaluating outcomes rather than simply reporting activities (Fredericks, Carman, & Birkland, 2002; Wholey, 2003). However, increased demands have not necessarily led to best practices in evaluation. Best practices in evaluation rarely occur for two main reasons: lack of general knowledge about what constitutes good evaluation practice on the part of those retaining evaluators, and the late stage in which evaluators are brought into the process.

Lack of Public Knowledge of Good Evaluation Practices

Very few organizational leaders or personnel at funding agencies have the training to recognize good evaluation practices. Although most funding applications for social (and other) programs do require applicants to include an evaluation plan, few allow a line item in the budget for evaluation work. This means that the program staff will be conducting their own evaluations. In addition, the expectations of what these evaluations should be are quite low in most applications. In my thirteen years running nonprofit social service organizations, most funding sources have been satisfied with an evaluation that amounts to little more than a client exit survey (e.g., "On a scale of one to ten, with ten being the highest, rate how satisfied you were with this service"). These kinds of exit surveys often translate into staff popularity contests, rather than actual reported changes in client behaviors, attitudes, or knowledge. In addition, program leaders also have to rely on the integrity of their staff in collecting these surveys. This type of evaluation offers no assurance whatsoever that a paper program will not result.

Even when the budget funds use of an internal or external evaluator, organizational and program leaders rarely have enough knowledge of best evaluation practices to select one with adequate training and experience. Many college instructors and other professionals supplement their incomes as research consultants. Although they may have letters after their names, they also may have no knowledge whatsoever of evaluation models, methods, sampling strategies, statistical or qualitative analysis, or how to write up findings. But because personnel from funding sources and organizations themselves usually have limited knowledge of evaluation, they will tend to trust the practices of those with the advanced degrees.

I recall a situation in which our firm was brought in to complete an evaluation of a project designed to bring resources to neighborhoods. The first evaluator, who was actually a tenured sociology professor, had produced a report that the program director believed did not represent his program in any way. As the director told me, "I don't even recognize this project in his writings." When we began work on the program, we accessed the data that this evaluator had collected. He had only gone to the high-level coalition meetings where various bureaucrats battled over which neighborhoods received which resources, and never went to the actual neighborhoods where the resources were being dispersed. His report described a dysfunctional program due to the infighting over neighborhood and resource selection. In our follow-up, we studied the linkages between decisions at the meetings and the resources brought to (and subsequently dispersed in) the neighborhoods. We also conducted pre- and posttest surveys of residents in the neighborhoods receiving new resources and residents in comparison neighborhoods, and found a number of outstanding results for the neighborhoods receiving the resources.

In addition to lacking actual skills and experience in evaluation, some evaluators follow trendy new evaluation genres that may be nice matches for their skills but may not necessarily be appropriate for addressing the evaluation questions that need to be answered. Most of the new genres are effective for specific types of evaluation and not for others. For example, a friend of mine who taught at a local university received a contract to evaluate a gang prevention program. She read available material on "fourth generation evaluation" (Guba & Lincoln, 1989)—a genre designed to explicate how program stakeholders interpret program features rather than focusing on measuring outcomes. Interpretive strategies are very valuable for many types of studies (and our firm uses this genre often in our evaluations, when the genre fits the research questions), but in this case the evaluation contract specified she was supposed to evaluate specific outcomes. With no training in quantitative methods, my friend produced an evaluation report that centered on stakeholders' interpretation of the word *gang*. The program leaders expressed a good deal of dissatisfaction with the product they received. This ended up being a case of the genre leading the evaluation rather than the need to assess an intervention's effectiveness guiding the process. Again, this type of evaluation offers no assurance that a paper program will not result.

A final issue relating to the general lack of knowledge of good evaluation practices is the assumption some organizational leaders have about the costs of evaluation. Most evaluation consultants or firms with relatively low overhead can do an effective one-time evaluation of a medium-sized program (25 to 100 clients) for between $10,000 and $20,000. However, most of the calls our firm receives are from people who believe an evaluation can be conducted for less than $500. I often talk to program leaders who urge us to take on a "minievaluation" for a few hundred dollars, and they sometimes tell us that we would not even have to visit the program site—we could just look over the program records they would send us and draw conclusions about the effectiveness of the program. In these cases I usually have a list of researchers I know who will do these minievaluations from paper products only, and the program can contact them. Had any of these researchers evaluated the PAY program, where all the case management files were falsified, the PAY program might have ended up with a positive evaluation. Again, this type of evaluation offers no assurance at all that a paper program will not result.

The public's lack of knowledge of good evaluation practices is also problematic as it relates to the following issue.

Late Stage in Which Evaluators Are Brought into the Process

In my experience, evaluators are almost never brought into the assessment process early enough—when a program is ready to begin or even when a specific program cycle is about to begin. Why? First, at Jill Florence Lackey & Associates, we have found a general lack of knowledge about when evaluations should be conducted. Because they lack good information on evaluation practices, most who contact us believe evaluations are to be conducted when the program cycle is ended or about to end. These ideas may come from the popular media, where public opinion and market research tend to follow the event (e.g., "In your opinion, which of the following responses best describes the President's State of the Union address?" "Which of these three products you have tasted had the best flavor?"). In addition, many program leaders first think about commissioning an evaluation when a funding cycle is about to end or when they are considering looking for a new funding source. Many of the potential evaluation sponsors that contact us have no idea that best evaluation practice unfolds when the evaluator is present in the program's planning and implementation stages.

In addition, few programs can support more than an occasional evaluation, particularly if an external research firm or consultant is conducting the evaluation. When an evaluation is commissioned, it is usually done for one of two reasons. First, program staff may desire the evaluation because they believe they have a strong program and want this confirmed by a professional evaluator. Rarely do paper programs emerge here. But often these programs have been running for years, sometimes decades, and it may be too late to make any improvements suggested by evaluation findings, as the components within the program may be too entrenched.

Second, someone other than program staff may desire an evaluation (e.g., the funding source, parent organization). Government-funded programs often require a substantial amount of evaluation work. At times a parent organization or funding source may want to document reasons for funding a new program component, changing or ending a program, or even terminating staff. In this set of circumstances, we do find paper programs. Unfortunately, again, the program may have been in operation for years and it may be too late to make changes that would help the program improve. When someone other than program staff has requested the evaluation, it is not uncommon to find staff who are hostile to members of the evaluation team, suspicious of motives for the evaluation, unwilling to hand over client names or program records, or unavailable for feedback sessions.

Many of these issues arose when Jill Florence Lackey & Associates conducted an evaluation of a family-counseling program in a middle-class neighborhood. We were contacted by the parent organization's administrator and asked to submit an evaluation plan and budget for a program that had been in operation for eight years. The administrator gave us a typed program description and a funding reapplication and requested an evaluation plan from those documents. We designed an evaluation using mixed methods and a quasi-experimental model, but the administrator immediately asked us to discard the comparison group, citing budgetary reasons. We advised her of the limitations we would face in findings without a comparison group and when the director held her ground, we added another data source to try and strengthen the overall design. Her motive in wanting the evaluation was curious, as we immediately encountered a program that was barely operational.

For starters, the overall purpose of the program was unclear. In program documents, staff discussed a needs assessment that had been conducted eight years ago in the neighborhood. The major finding of the assessment was the concern that residents expressed over the movement of gangs into the area, whose members were trying to recruit their children. Somehow from this identified need a program was developed to train parents to improve their parenting skills and end physical punishment of their children (not a finding in the needs assessment). In actuality, the program had begun as an effort to help youth resist negative peer pressure (especially from the gang members), but the program experienced early staff turnover, and the new staff had skills in parent counseling (particularly in preventing parental physical abuse), and gradually the program moved from a youth decision-making model to a parental counseling focus, with no demonstrated needs to support the change. When parents failed to sign up for the program's training and counseling sessions, the program staff went to the local community center to request referrals. Although the community center staff told them they did not have enough information to refer children and families to the program for poor parenting, they did refer children who they knew to be underachievers in school, which they said could reflect family issues at home. The program staff ostensibly then met with the children, discussed home issues with them, and visited the parents to urge them to sign up for their parenting classes and counsel them on parenting skills.

But over time the community center staff had grown impatient with the program, arguing that they needed to see more improvement in school performance of referred students if they were to continue to make the referrals. Thus, the administrator of the parent organization wanted us to develop pre- and posttest instruments that focused on school performance. Hence what we had was this convoluted model of a program that unfolded as follows: A needs assessment in this neighborhood demonstrated a need for a youth decision-making program to teach kids to avoid negative peers; a program model then followed that was supposed to prevent physical punishment of children; and this model would be evaluated with the expected outcomes that the children would improve academic performance. I pointed out the inconsistencies of this design to the organization's administrator, and she finally conceded that we should also collect data on good parenting practices (as this is what the program was attempting to accomplish). She did, however, insist on collecting data on the academic performance as well, even though there was not at the time any program activity that would have directly impacted the students' grades.

However, as we developed the instruments and began administering the pretest questionnaires to parents and children on a list of new referrals we received from the community center, we noticed a rather obvious situation: No program staff were at work. The program's director was on leave for personal reasons, the second-in-command was out on maternity leave, another staff member just stopped coming to work, and two staff had been hired that month to fill the void but had nothing to do because their supervisors were not available to train them. The new staff came to work every day and basically read magazines. This situation continued for nearly two months. We could not access any program records or other needed materials because we had no one to help us, and of course there were no activities to observe. This program was not evaluable, but we were under contract to collect and analyze data for them for nine months, regardless.

Two developments followed that also affected the evaluation. First, when we had completed our parent and child pretest surveys, we failed to find a single example of use of physical punishment in the self-reports of the children or the parents. The program was set up to treat a problem that apparently did not exist in this group. Second, the organization's administrator sought to find something for the two new staff to do. She telephoned the community center and workers there suggested the staff come in and tutor the student referrals who were having academic problems. They did—for nearly twelve weeks.

After several months the program's director returned, as did her second-in-command. Despite our findings that their referred clientele reported no cases of physical punishment, the staff continued to call on the parents, inviting them to come to their workshops on changing their parenting practices. Only two parents of the forty-five families that year came to the workshops. The staff ostensibly made home visits to the parents, although no member of the evaluation team was ever given access to these visits. The two new staff were taken away from their tutoring duties and trained to counsel parents at their homes. At the end of the program year, findings for parental practices showed virtually no change between the pre- and posttest periods in indicators of effective parenting, such as time parents spent with children, numbers of family discussions, types of corrective behavior, and numbers of family activities (all practices the staff said they focused on during counseling sessions). Yet the children showed significant improvements in academic performance, possibly due to the previously unplanned (and later terminated) tutoring delivered when the newly hired staff had nothing else to do.

The evaluation reports (oral and written) recommended that the program conduct a new needs assessment to refocus the program on actual needs of the families referred through the community center, and not on the interests and training of the staff. None of the program's staff came to our feedback sessions or read the final report, by their own admission. Furthermore, the organization's administrator who had commissioned the evaluation resigned from her position a month before the evaluation report was submitted. The new administrator told us that the evaluation had been commissioned because of a lack of fit between the program's staff and the administrator, and for that reason the staff had little commitment to the evaluation results (I assumed she meant that the former administrator was looking for negative evaluation results to justify some staff changes). Furthermore, the new administrator stated, the program had served the area for eight years and had a stable funding source, and the organization could risk losing that funding source if they changed the focus. Hence, we were confronted with a situation in which an evaluation was conducted for divisive reasons, years too late to have any serious impact on the program's shortcomings, and the results appeared to be ignored. We also did not know if the results were ever shared with any funding sources. Another paper product sat on a shelf gathering dust.

At this time, the reader may wonder if there actually might be circumstances that promote early engagement of evaluators. There are. It is more likely to occur in cases of internal evaluators. In some situations, very large organizations or institutions have their own evaluation staff. We have occasionally worked in collaborative relationships with internal evaluators and recognize that they are more likely to have access to the program during planning and implementation stages than external evaluators. On the other hand, we have found them less likely than external evaluators to have an influence over program leaders during feedback sessions. The lack of influence is sometimes due to the fact that the program director outranks or is equal in rank to the evaluator in the organization's bureaucracy. Torres, Preskill, and Piontek (1997) compared the satisfaction that both internal and external evaluators experienced in their communicating and reporting efforts and found lower satisfaction for the internal evaluators. The results, the authors argued, were probably mediated by "the political constraints and complexities they experience within organizations" (p. 119). In the four cases where we have worked collaboratively with internal evaluators, the internal people consistently turned to us to deliver news that program change was indicated, at any stage of the evaluation.

In terms of external evaluators, there are actually circumstances when they should be brought into the process very early, or so it would appear on paper. Some funding sources require an evaluation component built into the process from the program's onset. Not infrequently, governmental funding agencies mandate the evaluation component throughout the duration of supported programs, particularly when these programs are new, large, and time limited. Often these grants are given out to organizations that are trying an innovative approach to address some social problem (sometimes called a *demonstration project*). The idea here is that if the evaluation demonstrates the approach is effective, the organization is expected to use these findings to secure ongoing funding for the project.

But even here, the evaluator is rarely commissioned until long after the program has been implemented. Why? Sometimes this delay is the result of organizational policies. Many, if not most, large human service organizations have policies that mandate an RFP process for contracts with consultants or outside agencies when the contract exceeds a certain number of dollars. In some cases, an external evaluator may have even helped the organization secure the grant by writing the evaluation section of the proposal, and yet the actual contract is still sent out for bids. The process of developing an RFP, assembling a review committee, waiting for the proposals, selecting the evaluator, and negotiating the final contract typically takes longer than nine months. In addition, this process is usually treated with much lower priority than tasks such as hiring program staff, recruiting clients, and nurturing referral sources. Even if a highly competent evaluator is eventually engaged, a paper program may already be in the making, or poorly designed program components may already be embedded in program practices.

Not all organizations require competitive processes. Yet even here the start of the evaluation may be delayed. Our firm is often called upon to help an organization secure a grant by writing the required evaluation section. On occasion we are also brought in while the program is being planned to provide input into the process. But in at least three-quarters of the cases, we are asked to write the evaluation section of the proposal twenty-four hours or less before the proposal deadline. Whenever possible, we then set up a prefunding agreement with the organization that states that we will fulfill the evaluator's role, but that we also reserve the right to modify the evaluation plan later per input from additional stakeholders or when unanticipated circumstances arise. However, even in these cases, our firm is rarely notified when funding is secured. Programs lacking conscientious leadership often experience long delays in securing basic components to begin work on the programs, and delay notifying evaluators, possibly until they feel their programs are on track. But even the most conscientious, ethical program leaders are often overwhelmed with the start-up work of hiring staff, organizing collaborators, equipping the sites, and securing client referral sources; for this reason, they do not work with the evaluators from day one. The low priority given to immediate engagement of the evaluator is again related to lack of public knowledge of best evaluation practices. An evaluator brought in long after a new program is implemented offers no assurance that a paper program will not result.

EVALUATION FEEDBACK
AND WHY IT IS SO SELDOM USED

Use of evaluation depends in part on the level of participation of all stakeholders in the process (House, 2003). Stakeholders include program personnel, collaborators, and, above all, consumers of services.

Involving Stakeholders

Torres et al. (1997) found that the evaluator's use of clear language and ongoing interaction with the stakeholders (including clients/consumers) from the evaluation planning stage onward can strengthen the ultimate use of evaluation findings. In my experience, their findings were right on target. However, except for the use of clear language in evaluation (which evaluators can surely control), evaluators are almost completely dependent on the program leaders to provide access to stakeholders who could be involved in the process. We have had little success in drawing stakeholders beyond the program staff into the evaluation process, even though nearly all of our own contracts include a participatory clause requiring this.

When entering an evaluation context, only the program staff have the names and contact information relating to their clientele and other stakeholders: They must bring them to the table or provide the evaluation team with their names. When we attend the evaluation planning meetings, rarely does anyone appear other than personnel from the program or the parent organization. There are various reasons for this. At times program staff are overburdened with program start-up work and simply do not have the available hours to make contacts with stakeholders. At other times, program staff do invite stakeholders to the meetings but the stakeholders do not come. It also sometimes happens that the evaluator is brought into the program so late in the program cycle that there is no time to do anything but dash out a pretest instrument and administer it to consumers who may have already been receiving the intervention for weeks or months. At still other times, program staff simply ignore the participatory clauses in our contracts and never invite other stakeholders to the table.

Ideological misunderstandings surface over this issue as well. As mentioned previously, program leaders can misunderstand the purpose of involving other stakeholders in the evaluation process. They may fail to see that more informed and involved stakeholders (beyond program staff) ultimately lead to both better evaluations and better programs. Instead they sometimes express concerns that this could interfere with their own decision-making roles and the roles of the evaluator. Some have also argued that the more contact the evaluator has with stakeholders—particularly program clients—the less objective the evaluator would become. This particular concern is misapplied, as best evaluation practice will always draw conclusions from multiple sources of data and not from the subjective impressions of one or two evaluators. Stufflebeam (1999) describes evaluation objectivity in the following way:

> Objectivist evaluations are based on the theory that moral good is objective and independent of personal or merely human feelings. They are firmly grounded in ethical principles, strictly control bias or prejudice in seeking determinations of merit and worth, invoke and justify appropriate and (where they exist) established standards of merit and worth, obtain and validate findings from multiple sources, set forth and justify conclusions about the evaluand's merit and/or worth, report findings honestly and fairly to all right-to-know audiences, and subject the evaluation process and findings to independent assessments against the standards of the evaluation field. (p. 329)

I recall an episode in my earliest years as an evaluator when I was giving feedback to a group of program stakeholders. This was the first time the organization's administrator was present during the process. After the meeting, he called me into his office and asked why I was doing this. He said that in his day, evaluators maintained a distance from those they were studying to ensure objectivity. I explained that most of the evaluation literature today argued for participation of stakeholders in evaluation decisions and certainly in feedback on findings. He was unconvinced.

Later that month, I attended a conference set up by this program's governmental funding source. One of the workshops was for evaluators. The topic selected by the funding source was participatory evaluation, and the presenters argued vehemently for involvement of all stakeholders (including consumers) in evaluation decision making. I and others in the room listened intently, nodded in agreement, and at the end of the presentation raised our hands in unison. The general comments went something like the following. "You are preaching to

the choir here, and not the people you should be addressing." "We try
and try to do this and the program people do not invite these stakeholders to the table." "The program staff think we are supposed to be
completely detached from those we are studying, or we are unprofes-
sional." "Loss of objectivity comes when the program staff are able to
control the evaluation, not when you involve those that are supposed
to receive the service."

I learned a lesson from my early evaluation activities and added a
participatory clause in later evaluation contracts. However, our firm
still faces considerable constraints from program and organizational
staff over involvement of key stakeholders—whether the reasons are
ideological or other. Participation by stakeholders in the evaluation
process is needed for more reasons than strengthening the evaluation
component. The bottom line is this: All possible groups of participants should play active roles in evaluation, as the more stakeholders
know what the program is supposed to do and achieve, and subsequently what the evaluation data indicate the program is really doing
and achieving, the less chance there is of a paper program developing.

Ultimate Use of Evaluation

At times the participatory process is not an option. Some funding
sources mandate that evaluators of programs they support maintain
an external stance when conducting evaluation and even refrain from
giving feedback until the program (or program cycle) ends. Hence
there are times when the evaluator is fully constrained from implementing participatory processes. But even here it is possible to effect
change (when needed) at the end of the evaluation period when the
final report is submitted. A reader-friendly report with findings supported solidly by data and a good overall research design should generate some responses.

But are these reports even read, and if so, by whom? Nearly all of
the evaluation contracts that Jill Florence Lackey & Associates has
held came from the parent organizations of the programs to be evaluated. The evaluation contracts stipulate that a written report will be
submitted by a specific date, often corresponding to some program
funding cycle or effort to secure new funds. In nearly every case, the
sponsoring organization's policies limit the overall contract period to
not more than thirty days after the evaluation report is due. However,

in common evaluation practice, the evaluation firm or consultant allows for a thirty-day review period for program stakeholders to read the evaluation for accuracy and suggest modifications (we always state that the final version is determined by the evaluator). In approximately half the cases, we never receive a response from the sponsoring organization—even when the results are mainly positive. In other cases, we really only hear from leaders of the sponsoring organization or the director of the program that was evaluated—almost never do we receive responses from the staff who are actually responsible for operating the program.

These leaders have varying (sometimes conflicting) motives in their review of reports. Some appear to really want to improve program services, activities, and resources. This motivation becomes quite apparent when we hold evaluation contracts for multiple years and can see the way they use the findings to improve the program. Others appear to be more concerned with how the evaluation will look to their funding agencies or how it might potentially look to outside sources that could access the report. When either of the last two motivations emerge, those reviewing the report tend to go to great lengths to argue for language changes for every negative finding. In these situations, the use of the evaluation appears to be related more to public image and funding considerations than to actually improving the program.

The duration of the evaluation contracts further complicates the use issue. More often than not, any responses we receive are not submitted until the very end of the evaluation contract, leaving us no time to present findings to the stakeholder audiences. In these cases, we volunteer to attend follow-up meetings on our own time to review the findings, but if we are no longer under contract with the sponsoring organization, we must rely on them to call the meetings. Never once in our experience has such a follow-up meeting been called, even when the evaluation was overwhelmingly positive. In one instance, we evaluated a school-based program that was well implemented and went beyond its goals in meeting its anticipated outcomes, but did not receive strong support from school administration. We saw this as a perfect venue for presentation and discussion of findings with stakeholders, including student participants, teachers, and in particular the school administration. Despite repeated offers to present the findings (months after our contract expired), the program leaders never responded.

We have experienced better results providing feedback to program stakeholders when we hold multiyear evaluation contracts. In such cases, we usually call the meetings ourselves, and because we have been working with these stakeholders for longer periods of time, we have access to all the contact information and have a history of past work with them. Val de Vall and Bolas (1981) have argued that internal evaluators might also have better chances of getting their results to stakeholders (hence the evaluation findings used) because they have more ongoing communication with these stakeholders. In either case, the meetings can then result in action plans to address evaluation findings—whether they are modifying problems or celebrating successes.

However, in our experience these examples of follow-up on use of evaluation findings are rare. The bottom line is that the sponsoring organization nearly always holds control over how the evaluation findings get to the stakeholders—whether program leaders actually read the reports themselves, whether they hand out the reports or the shorter executive summaries to others, whether they require that program staff read the report, whether they call meetings to discuss findings, whether they invite the evaluator back to address stakeholder audiences, and whether they ever use any evaluation findings or recommendations to improve the program in any way. This is the bottom line that has been stressed throughout this book. The sponsoring organization's control over use of evaluation provides no assurance whatsoever that a paper program will not result.

AND YET . . .

The work of evaluation might appear to be rife with tension, political constraints, and frustrations. At times this is true. But in my experience, it is also rife with rewards. As has been stated repeatedly, most programs that we have evaluated have not been paper programs. In fact most of the programs have had strong, positive outcomes. Over the past three years, we have conducted seven evaluations, three of them multiyear. Of these, one was a paper program. This program was funded in full five years ago and still has not implemented even one of the services spelled out in the original proposal. One program implemented most of its activities, services, and resources and achieved over half of its intended outcomes. The other five were well implemented and to date have achieved all of their intended outcomes. Outstanding programs do indeed exist in a relative vacuum of accountability mechanisms.

Chapter 7

The Paper Program and the Future

As defined in Chapter 1, paper programs are social service programs that exist, for the most part, on paper only. They have formal documents that specify the services or other resources they are supposed to provide, and routine documentation suggests the programs are providing what they claim, but in reality they are providing none or a mere fraction of these services. My argument throughout this book is that paper programs—and to an even greater degree, paper coalitions—develop in an environment that lacks accountability mechanisms among groups and cultural institutions with stakes in the social service delivery system. Although demands for accountability have actually increased through government and private mandates, nearly all monitoring in this system uses written communication rather than face-to-face interaction. Paper reports in essence become the program.

Social programs often develop in a hegemonic environment that influences their funding, their implementation, and their accountability requirements all the way down the line. Ethical program staff who are both client centered and public centered almost invariably implement strong programs. But where staff performance is mixed or staff are diverted by other priorities, accountability mechanisms are ostensibly in place to refocus the effort. The social service delivery system has four possible major sources of accountability for programs: (1) the potential service consumers (e.g., clientele, general public), (2) the funding sources, (3) the program's sponsoring or parent organizations, and (4) program evaluators. One might even add the mass media to that list. But all of these are affected by their relative positions in the system. The theory of hegemony best explains the shifting relationships within this arrangement. Social programs are embedded in systems that include groups ranging from the least powerful con-

doi:10.1300/5556_07

99

sumers or potential consumers of services to very powerful government and corporate interests. Social services may not be a high priority for the more powerful interests, and the process of merely securing initial and ongoing financial backing for the programs involves hegemonic negotiations and co-optation.

The theory of hegemony derives from the recognition that government and other dominant interests cannot enforce control over any subordinate groups without these groups yielding a limited consent (Gramsci, 1971). Dominant groups in capitalist societies rule through power blocs, or special purpose alliances, but subordinate formations also play roles in the development of policies and ideologies. Social service organizations or advocacy groups may negotiate their way into these alliances and get their interests represented. For example, the nonprofit parent organization of the No-Place-Like-Home program saw an opportunity to implement a program for the homeless by finding a legislator that would propose legislation to fund the proposed program. The legislator had a day shelter in his district with potential homeless voters and collaborated with the homeless themselves, advocates for them, the nonprofit organization, and other legislators. This newly created alliance was able to achieve its aims, and the proposed program was funded and implemented. A similar situation occurred with Project United-Are-We. As a major medical complex was seeing more victims of violence in their emergency rooms, they partnered with community groups, held press conferences, and also helped form an alliance of legislators and other potential funding sources to fund a program to work with the victims.

What kind of active interest do the more powerful members of these alliances maintain in the programs, once funded? The case studies presented here suggest that the interest is limited. For example, although major political, institutional, and business leaders sat on the original REDUCE coalition, no members of this group called for action when the coalition was presented with early evaluation findings revealing lack of program implementation. Leaders of a county social services department implemented very few of their promised services to increase the health of their teens, then failed to even mention the multiyear/multimillion-dollar grant they held when interviewed by a reporter on the alarming news that this county had just advanced to number one in numbers of unhealthy teens. Personnel at large funding agencies (including government centers) routinely ignored evaluation findings, even when special efforts were made to alert the agencies to program shortcomings.

Co-optation abounded at multiple levels in the system, often having the effect of reducing incentives to impose accountability mechanisms that could expose paper programs. In our firm's experience evaluating programs, public funding agencies, attempting to justify their programs (and actually their existence) to lawmaking bodies, sought optimistic reports of the initiatives they supported. Private funding agencies needed to show their large donors that they were accomplishing much with their dollars. At times private funding agencies ran their own social service coalitions, resulting in a near-perfect co-optation of member organizations that they funded in other venues. Citizen activists failed to report social program failings run by large bureaucracies for fear of losing important linkages. The parent organizations of social programs also had weak incentives to track down shortcomings as they worked to maintain reputations of running sound programs to their funding sources and powerful collaborators. To further compound the issue, program evaluators are habitually funded and controlled by the very organizations they are supposed to be evaluating. The monitoring functions of evaluators are further constrained by the lack of public knowledge about good evaluation practices, the late stages at which evaluators are brought into the monitoring process (when paper programs may already be in the works), and the lack of use of evaluation findings by all stakeholders up and down the system.

At the local program level, many staff discuss commitment to clients (and many clearly demonstrate this commitment), but the mandated requirements for reporting tend to focus on printed products rather than client-staff relations. This mismatch between expressed ideals and daily practices is a core element in Bourdieu's (1977) theory of practice. Bourdieu argued that dispositions and embedded practices, rather than ideals, tend to guide human behavior. Although the practices may have emerged as adaptations to environmental factors, over time the factors may be forgotten, and the practices continue with minimal reflection. One of these practices that emerged is the tendency to replace the real with a representation of the real (Baudrillard, 1994). In human services, written documentation has always been necessary for communicating with other staff to maintain a history of the services or resources that have been provided, and obviously because no one can be present to monitor every transaction—and the documentation has to be the next best thing. The problems begin when the representation of the transaction becomes the "proof" of the transaction, and ultimately when the representation replaces the transaction itself, which has gradually become the norm in social services. Funding sources for programs usually require written reports of program operations and expenditures, but funding personnel seldom conduct site visits to determine whether these services are actually provided. This process has become a virtual reality of accountability mechanisms.

Examples of paper programs emerge in this environment. The staff of PAY, Programs on the Plains, REDUCE, and TeenHealth worked in a system where the representations of programs became the proof that these programs existed. Staff progress reports, in most cases, had replaced on-site monitoring. The staff were professionals with social service education and training and years of experience in human service organizations. They had skills in creating carefully crafted proposals and reapplications, building program images through computer-generated flowcharts and conceptual models, supplying boards and coalitions with sizable reports, designing public relations documents, issuing press releases of program activities, creating program Web pages, giving formal presentations (even through digital media), and producing timely reports to monitoring agencies. They left paper trails sufficient to satisfy parent organizations, coalition partners, funding agencies, and—in the case of PAY—even organizational audits. In actuality, we found that programs that exist in planning processes only—that barely exist beyond their paper representations—can continue to draw millions of funding dollars for years and years.

In our experience, the amazing part of the story is that most social service programs are not paper programs despite the dearth of accountability mechanisms. Most that our firm evaluated were well-implemented and efficiently run programs that evaluated positively. Some of these programs were modeled in such a way that staff discretion was nearly impossible. They were solidly publicized, offered standardized services, and had stable program sites where consumers could gather in mass (as opposed to being served individually). But the "one size fits all" program rarely addressed issues involving more complex human and social problems. The other exceptional programs stood out for their ethics-based leadership—they had personnel with a private sense of duty toward clients, a public sense of duty toward the general community, and attributes of sacrifice, a voice of conscience, and assurance of competence at all service levels. When ethics-based leaders managed to remain in their positions for long periods of time (not something likely to happen often in unstable funding and political environments), they ultimately helped create a subculture of client-centered service by retaining staff with their value systems and easing out staff with alternative philosophies.

However, even in these nearly ideal environments, co-optation abounded, often preventing program staff from protecting their services and their consumers. When a powerful political leader maligned the PC&C program, the program's director was not allowed to defend the program's reputation in the media because the political leader sat on the board of the parent organization. When the urban garden staff were about to lose their gardening land when the city considered a motion to sell the land to developers, they could not help their multilingual/multicultural clients organize against the motion because the city controlled other resources the program needed.

The ultimate losers in the paper programs and the co-opted relationships have been the consumers and potential consumers of social services—those who currently occupy the least powerful place in the hegemonic relationships. In our experience they were sometimes used to secure initial funding, but after that played almost no role in ensuring that the services were offered in accordance with the program's promises. Program leaders who had very strong ethics tended to put the interests of the service consumers and the general public before others in the social service delivery system, but they did this out of personal dispositions as opposed to systemic requirements. Clearly one conclusion that must be drawn from these case studies is that the consumers need to be more than just means to ends in helping draw funds for social service providers. They need to be the ends themselves throughout the process, and to achieve this aim they must be integrally involved in ensuring that programs are implemented per their paper promises and accountability mechanisms are in place. Another group that has been cut out of the process in many ways and that must be integrally involved is lower-level staff in the programs themselves.

A VENUE FOR CHANGE

Sue Golding (1988) argued that Gramsci's view of hegemony made revolutionary change possible. Groups from subordinate formations could also enter into hegemonic relationships and negotiate power. In his research, Fiske (1993) stressed the potential power of bottom-up local groups (emphasizing consumers) in confronting the top-down imperializing power in hegemonic relationships. There is a history of this in human services. In the past, disabled groups such as the blind, the mentally ill, and their families have been successful at effecting policy changes on disability rights, self-determination, and freedom of choice. Much of this work has fallen under the category of consumer movements that began in the United States as early as the National Consumer's League in 1899 and have continued to the present—today strongly influenced by the work of Ralph Nader (Maclachlan & Trentmann, 2004).

Much of Nader's success came through development of public interest research groups (PIRGs) that were founded in colleges, universities, and other community venues. Scores of these PIRGs have dealt with consumer issues such as fraud in auto repair, subway service, dental health, water pollution, banking and credit, property tax assessments, and toxic waste, to name but a few. They have collected dues from members and through this channel have been able to engage staff and consultants with relevant skills and education, such as community organizing, science, and the law. Through the work of staff, consultants, members, and other volunteers, many of these PIRGs have been able to collect and disseminate information about local products and services, monitor the producers, and hold them accountable to the public (Bollier, 1991).

Consumers and potential consumers of services, lower-level program staff who want to improve their programs, and good citizens could develop their own local PIRGs on local social services. Members could inform the public on what social services exist and what the services' official documents indicate they are to provide, and in the process develop some forms of accountability mechanisms. Examples could include providing forums for consumer complaints; developing a hierarchy for circulating these complaints (such as notifying the parent organization, the program's funding sources, appropriate government agencies and elected representatives, and other mass media); effecting policy changes to tighten accountability mechanisms; and maintaining "report cards" on programs that are well implemented based on their own experiences, site visits, or attempts to access service. Another function might be working with local social and human service organizations and relevant university departments (such as social work, organizational leadership, public health, social welfare) to enhance the emphasis on ethics-based leadership in social programs (see Manning, 2003).

One element needed to hold services accountable is a way to decrease the control that programs (or their parent organizations) have over their evaluators. Funding sources working with potential program consumers might commission evaluators or conduct the evaluations themselves, if they have staff with training in best evaluation practices. The consumer groups forming PIRGs might in certain cases commission evaluations with their expert staff or consultants. They might play strong roles in the selection of evaluators, help select the success indicators the evaluators need to assess, be the source of review and use of evaluation findings, educate program personnel on best evaluation practices, or, at minimum, serve as mediators between the evaluation sponsors and the evaluators. Evaluation needs consumers and potential consumers to be involved in every stage of the process to ensure that findings are reliable and relevant to the very people the program is supposed to be helping.

How might this process expand actual use of evaluation findings? One role of the consumer groups forming PIRGs might be to identify the funding sources of the programs being evaluated and alert the funders to both program strengths and weaknesses that emerged from the findings. If the PIRGs remain steadfast in the goal of representing the welfare of consumers and potential consumers of services, many funding agencies might begin imposing sanctions on their funded programs with weak evaluation outcomes. All transactions of the PIRGs could be covered on the groups' Web sites.

BEFORE PUTTING THIS BOOK DOWN

Before closing the book on the paper program, I would like the reader to consider one last point. Paper programs affect everyone. The reader might have scrutinized every case study in these chapters and noted that the consumers of the highlighted programs were youthful offenders, unhealthy adults, drug addicts, victims of violence, overweight teens, hungry immigrants, unemployed urbanites, the homeless, underachieving children, or ex-felons. The reader might think, "Well, this is interesting information, but not terribly relevant to my life." The reader might also wonder if this motley group together with low-level program staff would really band together in any kind of consumer movement. The truth is this: Any consumer movement trying to hold these social programs accountable must include the general public as well as consumers of specific services. The public's interest is a great part of this accountability process. Members of the general public are the victims of crime if the offending youths or ex-felons reoffend. Members of the general public pay higher insurance premiums when social programs that are supposed to be improving the health of communities do not do their jobs. Members of the general public have higher tax bills when the crime rate increases, or unemployment increases, or immigrants need food stamps to feed their families. Consumer empowerment encompasses the general public. This is an issue that needs to be addressed, and addressed by and for the citizenry.

References

Chapter 1

Baudrillard, J. (1994). *Simulacra and simulation* (S.G. Glaser, Trans.). Ann Arbor: University of Michigan Press.

Bourdieu, P. (1977). *Outline of a theory of practice* (R. Nice, Trans.). Cambridge: Cambridge University Press. (Original work published 1972.)

Canclini, N.G. (1995). *Hybrid cultures: Strategies for entering and leaving modernity.* Minneapolis: University of Minnesota Press.

Gramsci, A. (1971). *Selections from the prison notebooks* (Q. Hoare & G.N. Smith, Ed. and Trans.). New York: International Publishers.

Harvey, C. (1998). Defining excellence in human service organizations. *Administration in Social Work, 22*(1), 33-45.

Jameson, F. (1984). Postmodernism, or the cultural logic of late capitalism. *New Left Review, 146,* 53-92.

Manning, S.S. (2003). *Ethical leadership in human services: A multi-dimensional approach.* Boston: Pearson Education.

Martin, L.L., & Kettner, P.M. (1997). Performance measurement: The new accountability. *Administration in Social Work, 21*(1), 17-29.

Rapp, C.A., & Poertner, J. (1992). *Social administration: A client-centered approach.* New York: Longman.

Chapter 2

Aiken, S.S., & West, S.G. (1990). Invalidity of true experiments: Self-report pretest biases. *Evaluation Review, 14*(4), 374-390.

Baudrillard, J. (1994). *Simulacra and simulation* (S.G. Glaser, Trans.). Ann Arbor: University of Michigan Press.

Cousins, J.B., & Earl, J. (1995). The case for participatory evaluation. *Educational Evaluation and Policy Analysis, 14,* 397-418.

Derber, C., Schwartz, W.A., & Magrass, Y. (1990). *Power in the highest degree: Professionals and the rise of a new mandarin order.* New York: Oxford University Press.

Fetterman, D.M. (1994). Empowerment evaluation. *Evaluation Practice, 15*(1), 1-15.

Fetterman, D.M. (1996). Introduction and overview. In D.M. Fetterman, S.J. Kaftarian, & A. Wandersman (Eds.), *Empowerment evaluation: Knowledge and*

doi:10.1300/5556_08

tools for self-assessment and accountability (pp. 1-15). Thousand Oaks, CA: Sage.

Friedson, E. (1984). Are professions necessary? In T. Haskell (Ed.), *The authority of experts: Studies in history and theory* (pp. 3-27). Bloomington: Indiana University Press.

Guba, E.G., & Lincoln, Y.S. (1989). *Fourth generation evaluation.* Newbury Park, CA: Sage.

House, E.R. (2003). Stakeholder bias. In C.A. Christie (Ed.), *The practice-theory relationship in evaluation* (New Directions for Evaluation, No. 97). San Francisco: Jossey-Bass.

Howard, G.S. (1980). Response-shift bias: A problem in evaluating interventions with pre/post self-reports. *Evaluation Review, 4*(1), 93-106.

Kirschner, D.S. (1986). *The paradox of professionalism: Reform and public service in urban America, 1900-1940.* New York: Greenwood Press.

Lackey, J.F., Moberg, D.P., & Balistrieri, M. (1997). By whose standards? Reflections on empowerment evaluation and grassroots groups. *Evaluation Practice, 18*(2), 137-146.

Meyer, J.M., & Rowan, B. (1977). Institutional organizations: Formal structure as myth and ceremony. *American Journal of Sociology, 83*(2), 340-363.

Patton, M.Q. (1978). *Utilization-focused evaluation.* Beverly Hills, CA: Sage.

Patton, M.Q. (1997). *Utilization-focused evaluation: The new century text.* Thousand Oaks, CA: Sage.

Perrow, C. (1972). *Complex organizations: A critical essay.* Glenview, IL: Scott, Foresman and Co.

Scriven, M. (1997). Empowerment evaluation examined. *Evaluation Practice, 18*(2), 165-175.

Shadish, W.R., Cook, T.D., & Leviton, L.C. (1991). Good theory for social program evaluation. In W.R. Shadish, T.D. Cook, & L.C. Leviton (Eds.), *Foundations of program evaluation: Theories of practice* (pp. 36-67). Newbury Park, CA: Sage.

Tax, S. (1958). The Fox project. *Human Organization, 17,* 17-19.

Weiss, C.H. (1998). *Evaluation: Methods for studying programs and policies* (2nd ed.). Upper Saddle River, NJ: Prentice Hall.

Whyte, W.F. (Ed.). (1991). *Participatory action research.* Newbury Park, CA: Sage.

Chapter 3

Bourdieu, P. (1977). *Outline of a theory of practice* (R. Nice, Trans.). Cambridge: Cambridge University Press. (Original work published 1972.)

Dluhly, M.J. (1990). *Building coalitions in the human services.* Newbury Park, CA: Sage.

Perrow, C. (1972). *Complex organizations: A critical essay.* Glenview, IL: Scott, Foresman and Co.

Richards, R.W. (1996). *Building partnerships: Educating health professionals for the communities they serve.* San Francisco: Jossey-Bass.

Chapter 4

Bonk, K., Griggs, H., & Tynes, E. (1999). *The Jossey-Bass guide to strategic communications for nonprofits.* San Francisco: Jossey-Bass.

Bourdieu, P. (1977). *Outline of a theory of practice* (R. Nice, Trans.). Cambridge: Cambridge University Press. (Original work published 1972.)

Fetterman, D.M. (1994). Empowerment evaluation. *Evaluation Practice, 15*(1), 1-15.

Frost, C. (2002). *Reporting for journalists.* London: Routledge.

Gans, H. (1979). *Deciding what's news: A study of CBS Evening News, NBC Nightly News, Newsweek, and Time.* New York: Vintage Books.

Goldman, R., & Rajagopal, A. (1991). *Mapping hegemony: Television news coverage of industrial conflict.* Norwood, NJ: Ablex.

Gramsci, A. (1971). *Selections from the prison notebooks* (Q. Hoare & G.N. Smith, Ed. and Trans.). New York: International Publishers.

Hall, S. (1977). Culture, the media, and the "ideological effect." In J. Curran, M. Gurevitch, & J. Woollacott (Eds.), *Mass communication and society* (pp. 315-348). London: Arnold.

Chapter 5

Manning, S.S. (2003). *Ethical leadership in human services: A multi-dimensional approach.* Boston: Pearson Education.

National Association of Social Workers. (1996). *NASW code of ethics.* Washington, DC: NASW.

Reamer, F. (1998). The evolution of social work ethics. *Social Work, 43*(6), 488-500.

Wheatley, M., & Kellner-Rogers, M. (1999). *A simpler way.* San Francisco: Berrett-Koehler.

Chapter 6

American Evaluation Association. (1995). *Guiding principles for evaluators* (New Directions for Evaluation, No. 66). San Francisco: Jossey-Bass.

Bernstein, D.J., Whitsett, M.D., & Mohan, R. (2002). Addressing sponsor and stakeholder needs in the evaluation authorizing environment: Trends and implications. In R. Mohan, D.J. Bernstein, & M.D. Whitsett (Eds.), *Responding to sponsors and stakeholders in complex evaluation environments* (New Directions for Evaluation, No. 95, pp. 89-99). San Francisco: Jossey-Bass.

Crane, J. (1998). Building on success. In J. Crane (Ed.), *Social programs that work* (pp. 1-15). New York: Russell Sage Foundation.

Creswell, J.W. (2003). *Research design: Qualitative, quantitative, and mixed methods approaches* (2nd ed.). Thousand Oaks, CA: Sage.

Fetterman, D.M. (1996). Introduction and overview. In D.M. Fetterman, S.J. Kaftarian, & A. Wandersman (Eds.), *Empowerment evaluation: Knowledge and tools for self-assessment and accountability* (pp. 1-15). Thousand Oaks, CA: Sage.

Fredericks, K.A., Carman, J.G., & Birkland, T.A. (2002). Program evaluation in a challenging authorizing environment: Intergovernmental and interorganizational factors. In R. Mohan, D.J. Bernstein, & M.D. Whitsett (Eds.), *Responding to sponsors and stakeholders in complex evaluation environment* (New Directions for Evaluation, No. 95, pp. 5-21). San Francisco: Jossey-Bass.

Guba, E.G., & Lincoln, Y.S. (1989). *Fourth generation evaluation*. Newbury Park, CA: Sage.

House, E.R. (2003). Stakeholder bias. In C.A. Christie (Ed.), *The practice-theory relationship in evaluation* (New Directions for Evaluation, No. 97, pp. 53-56). San Francisco: Jossey-Bass.

Owen, J.M., & Rogers, P.J. (1999). *Program evaluation: Forms and approaches*. London: Sage.

Patton, M.Q. (1997). *Utilization-focused evaluation: The new century text*. Thousand Oaks, CA: Sage.

Rossi, P.H., Freeman, H.E., & Lipsey, M.W. (1999). *Evaluation: A systematic approach* (6th ed.). Thousand Oaks, CA: Sage.

Rutman, L. (1980). *Planning useful evaluations*. Beverly Hills, CA: Sage.

Scriven, M. (1983). Evaluation ideologies. In G. Madaus, M. Scriven, & D. Stufflebeam (Eds.), *Evaluation models: Viewpoints on educational and human services evaluation* (pp. 229-260). Boston: Kluwer-Nijhoff.

Stufflebeam, D.L. (1994). Empowerment evaluation, objectivist evaluation, and evaluation standards: Where the future of evaluation should not go and where it needs to go. *Evaluation Practice, 15*(3), 321-338.

Torres, R.T., Preskill, H.S., & Piontek, M.E. (1997). Communicating and reporting: Practices and concerns of internal and external evaluators. *Evaluation Practice, 18*(3), 105-125.

Val de Vall, M., & Bolas, C.A. (1981, June). External vs. internal social policy researchers. *Knowledge: Creation, Diffusion, Utilization, 2,* 461-481.

Weiss, C.H. (1987). Where politics and evaluation research meet. In D.J. Palumbo (Ed.), *The politics of program evaluation* (pp. 47-70). Newbury Park, CA: Sage.

Wholey, J.S. (2003). Improving performance and accountability: Responding to emerging management challenges. In S.I. Donaldson & M. Scriven (Eds.), *Evaluating social programs and problems* (pp. 43-61). Mahwah, NJ: Lawrence Erlbaum Associates.

Chapter 7

Baudrillard, J. (1994). *Simulacra and simulation* (S.G. Glaser, Trans.). Ann Arbor: University of Michigan Press.

Bollier, D. (1991). *Citizen action and other big ideas: A history of Ralph Nader and the modern consumer movement.* Washington, DC: Center for Study of Responsive Law.

Bourdieu, P. (1977). *Outline of a theory of practice* (R. Nice, Trans.). Cambridge: Cambridge University Press. (Original work published 1972.)

Fiske, J. (1993). *Power plays/power works.* London: Verso.

Golding, S. (1988). The concept of the philosophy of praxis in the *Quaderni* of Antonio Gramsci. In C. Nelson & L. Grossberg (Eds.), *Marxism and the interpretation of culture* (pp. 543-563). Urbana: University of Illinois Press.

Gramsci, A. (1971). *Selections from the prison notebooks* (Q. Hoare & G.N. Smith, Ed. and Trans.). New York: International Publishers.

Maclachlan, P., & Trentmann, F. (2004). Civilising markets: Traditions of consumer politics in twentieth-century Britain, Japan, and the United States. In M. Bevir & F. Trentmann (Eds.), *Markets in historical contexts: Ideas and politics in the modern world* (pp. 170-201). Cambridge: Cambridge University Press.

Manning, S.S. (2003). *Ethical leadership in human services: A multi-dimensional approach.* Boston: Pearson Education.

Index

doi:10.1300/5556_09

Order a copy of this book with this form or online at:
http://www.haworthpress.com/store/product.asp?sku=5556

ACCOUNTABILITY IN SOCIAL SERVICES
The Culture of the Paper Program

_____ in hardbound at $39.95 (ISBN-13: 978-0-7890-2374-2; ISBN-10: 0-7890-2374-1)

_____ in softbound at $14.95 (ISBN-13: 978-0-7890-2375-9; ISBN-10: 0-7890-2375-X)

Or order online and use special offer code HEC25 in the shopping cart.

COST OF BOOKS_____

POSTAGE & HANDLING_____
*(US: $4.00 for first book & $1.50
for each additional book)*
*(Outside US: $5.00 for first book
& $2.00 for each additional book)*

SUBTOTAL_____

IN CANADA: ADD 7% GST_____

STATE TAX_____
*(NJ, NY, OH, MN, CA, IL, IN, PA, & SD
residents, add appropriate local sales tax)*

FINAL TOTAL_____
*(If paying in Canadian funds,
convert using the current
exchange rate, UNESCO
coupons welcome)*

☐ **BILL ME LATER:** (Bill-me option is good on
US/Canada/Mexico orders only; not good to
jobbers, wholesalers, or subscription agencies.)
☐ Check here if billing address is different from
shipping address and attach purchase order and
billing address information.

Signature_____

☐ **PAYMENT ENCLOSED: $_____**

☐ **PLEASE CHARGE TO MY CREDIT CARD.**

☐ Visa ☐ MasterCard ☐ AmEx ☐ Discover
☐ Diner's Club ☐ Eurocard ☐ JCB

Account # _____

Exp. Date_____

Signature_____

Prices in US dollars and subject to change without notice.

NAME_____

INSTITUTION_____

ADDRESS_____

CITY_____

STATE/ZIP_____

COUNTRY_____ COUNTY (NY residents only)_____

TEL_____ FAX_____

E-MAIL_____

May we use your e-mail address for confirmations and other types of information? ☐ Yes ☐ No
We appreciate receiving your e-mail address and fax number. Haworth would like to e-mail or fax special
discount offers to you, as a preferred customer. **We will never share, rent, or exchange your e-mail address
or fax number.** We regard such actions as an invasion of your privacy.

Order From Your Local Bookstore or Directly From
The Haworth Press, Inc.
10 Alice Street, Binghamton, New York 13904-1580 • USA
TELEPHONE: 1-800-HAWORTH (1-800-429-6784) / Outside US/Canada: (607) 722-5857
FAX: 1-800-895-0582 / Outside US/Canada: (607) 771-0012
E-mail to: orders@haworthpress.com

For orders outside US and Canada, you may wish to order through your local
sales representative, distributor, or bookseller.
For information, see http://haworthpress.com/distributors

(Discounts are available for individual orders in US and Canada only, not booksellers/distributors.)
PLEASE PHOTOCOPY THIS FORM FOR YOUR PERSONAL USE.
http://www.HaworthPress.com   BOF06